UROLOGICAL CANCER

UROLOGICAL CANCER
A Practical Guide to Management

LESLIE EF MOFFAT

Grampian University Hospitals NHS Trust
University of Aberdeen
UK

MARTIN DUNITZ

© 2002 Martin Dunitz Ltd, a member of the Taylor & Francis group

First published in the United Kingdom in 2002
by Martin Dunitz Ltd, The Livery House, 7–9 Pratt Street, London NW1 0AE

Tel.:   +44 (0) 20 74822202
Fax.:   +44 (0) 20 72670159
E-mail: info@dunitz.co.uk
Website: http://www.dunitz.co.uk

Although every effort has been made to ensure that all owners of copyright material have been acknowledged in this publication, we would be glad to acknowledge in subsequent reprints or editions any omissions brought to our attention.

Although every effort has been made to ensure that drug doses and other information are presented accurately in this publication, the ultimate responsibility rests with the prescribing physician. Neither the publishers nor the authors can be held responsible for errors or for any consequences arising from the use of information contained herein. For detailed prescribing information or instructions on the use of any product or procedure discussed herein, please consult the prescribing information or instructional material issued by the manufacturer.

A CIP record for this book is available from the British Library.

ISBN 1-84184-190-0

Distributed in the USA by
Fulfilment Center
Taylor & Francis
7625 Empire Drive
Florence, KY 41042, USA
Toll Free Tel.: +1 800 634 7064
E-mail: cserve@routledge_ny.com

Distributed in Canada by
Taylor & Francis
74 Rolark Drive
Scarborough, Ontario M1R 4G2, Canada
Toll Free Tel.: +1 877 226 2237
E-mail: tal_fran@istar.ca

Distributed in the rest of the world by
ITPS Limited
Cheriton House
North Way
Andover, Hampshire SP10 5BE, UK
Tel.: +44 (0)1264 332424
E-mail: reception@itps.co.uk

Composition by Wearset Ltd, Boldon, Tyne and Wear

Printed and bound in Great Britain by Biddles Ltd, Guildford and King's Lynn.

To the ladies in my life: Elaine, Lisa, Vikki and Julia

'From the inability to let well alone; from too much zeal for the new and contempt for what is old; from putting knowledge before wisdom, science before art and cleverness before common sense; from treating patients as cases and from making the cure of the disease more grievous than it's endurance, good Lord deliver us.'

Sir Robert Hutchinson, Physician.
Murray JG. A Gentleman Publishers Commonplace Book. London.
John Murray. 1996.

Contents

Preface

Urological cancers are remarkable common and yet rarely fail to get headline acknowledgement. In the United Kingdom, as with much of the Western world, prostate cancer is increasing in incidence and also in prevalence. Prostate cancer is now the second leading cancer cause of death in the United Kingdom.

Testicular cancers are increasing in incidence and bladder tumours are increasing in women, possibly due to increased smoking. Many advances in cancer treatment have occurred in urology. It was the first speciality to identify industrial cancers. We have had excellent disease markers in the form of acid phosphatase and more recently prostate-specific antigen. Chemotherapy transformed survival in testicular cancer. Cytokines were demonstrated to have activity in renal cell cancer and intravesical BCG treatment has played a significant role in the management of bladder cancer.

There is a constant need to update books and concise texts encompassing the entire field of urological oncology are rare.

This book has been written to provide a concise overview of urological cancers and aimed primarily at medical staff, SPRs and PAMs involved in the urological oncology teams in both surgery, radiotherapy and oncology.

Salient facts are highlighted, along with case histories to illustrate important points. Although controversy is not avoided, the text outlines standard management in the U.K., Europe and North America.

This book may also be of interest to a wider public. Significant details have been given where necessary and a comprehensive reading list is included.

Leslie Moffat
Aberdeen, 2002

Acknowledgements

I would like to record my gratitude to Miss Linda Smith for her help with typing the manuscript.

Ms Maìre Collins has provided much encouragement at the inception and the support of Clive Lawson in editing and Alan Burgess in publishing is gratefully acknowledged.

My colleagues, Dr JD Bissett, Dr M Brooks, Mr N Cohen, Dr D Culligan, Dr V Duddalwar, Dr A Hutcheon, Mr SF Mishriki, Mr J N'Dow, Professor F Odds, Mr S Swami and Dr E Tiornan, as are Ms F Chilcot and Dr A Ritchie of the John Mallard Scottish PET Centre, are gratefully acknowledged, as is the help from the Department of Medical Illustration, University of Aberdeen, particularly Zoe Kaka, Nigel Lukins and Bruce Mireylees. Professor Malcolm Mason has made many helpful comments as has Dr Graeme Murray who has also reviewed the pathology sections.

Despite the above help, any errors are of course mine.

I would also like to record my gratitude to the many patients over the years, who have suffered their illnesses with a dignity and courage, which continues to provide a stimulus to those of us who have the privilege of attending them.

1

Introduction: urological cancer and the environment

Man is more the product of his environment than of his genetic endowment. The health of human beings is determined not by their race but by the conditions under which they live.[1]

Rene Jules Dubos

In this heady era of gene research and discovery, it is sobering to realise that environment continues to interact with the individual and their genes.

In the Western World, mortality from many causes such as infection has generally decreased. People are living longer and this has had the effect of increasing mortality from cancer: in particular, cancers of older people such as prostate cancer.[2]

CANCER REGISTRIES

Many nations around the world maintain cancer registries whose primary aim is to measure the number of new cases of cancer per year per 100,000 persons: this is known as the incidence rate. The number of deaths per 100,000 persons per year is the mortality rate. By determining the proportion of patients who are alive at some point after their diagnosis of cancer, a survival rate can be computed.

Cancer incidence is monitored by population-based tumour registries. Many countries are unable to measure these statistics and, even in the United States, the registries do not monitor the entire population. Incidence data from population-based registries are compiled by the International Agency for Research on Cancer

(IARC), as part of the World Health Organization (WHO). In order to compare like with like, various rates are age-adjusted to the world standard population. The reason for this is to eliminate differences in rates when the population of one country has a different age distribution from that of another country. These data can then be used in planning health services.

Death rates can be compared between different countries, but mortality rates are influenced by a number of factors, such as different incidence rates, different distributions of prognostic factors, such as stage, and of course differences in survival rates.

SEER

In the United States in 1973, the National Cancer Institute (NCI) began the Surveillance, Epidemiology and End Results (SEER) programme, to estimate cancer incidence and patient survival in the United States.

They collect cancer incidence data in nine geographical areas, with a combined population of approximately 9.6% of the entire US population.

Trends

Two measures to evaluate trends are given:

1. the estimated annual per cent change (EAPC)
2. the per cent change.

The EAPC is calculated by linear regression fit through the logarithms of the annual rates. The per cent change is calculated between the average of the 1973–74 rates, and the average of the 1990 and 1991 rates.

COMPARISON OF CANCER INCIDENCE IN DIFFERENT COUNTRIES

It is now possible to compare rates for different cancers between different countries and an overall calculation of cancer risk can be tabulated (Table 1.1). It can be seen from the table that we all have a varying risk of various types of cancer. It is difficult to speculate why some groups should have such an increased incidence compared with others. The incidences have been standardised with respect to age to make the statistics more meaningful.

To attempt an understanding of cancer, it is necessary to understand in part the role of the gene and the role of cellular control of cell division as well as appreciating the role of external influences on the cell.

ENVIRONMENTAL CAUSES OF CANCER

External factors

Cancer may have many causes but environmental factors are important in certain cancers. Percivall Pott (1714–88) wrote the first description of an occupational cancer of the scrotum in 1775.[4]

Ludwig Rehn (1849–1930) described in 1895 the frequent discovery of cancer of the bladder in men employed in the aniline dye industry.[5] These observations led the way to modern

---

Table 1.1 International comparisons of incidence rates of all cancers. Age-standardised incidence rates per 100,000 person-years at risk (World standard population) for selected countries or registries; ranked; by sex: period 1988–92.

Males	Females
US, SEER: White (1988–92) 454.6	New Zealand: Non-Maori 274.6
France, Bas-Rhin 394.0	US, SEER: White (1988–92) 271.6
Germany, Saarland 316.6	Denmark 261.6
Switzerland 312.2	Scotland 256.8
Australia, Victoria 307.1	Australia, Victoria 239.3
Scotland 306.2	France, Bas-Rhin 229.3
New Zealand: Non-Maori 290.4	Sweden 228.5
Netherlands (1989–92) 288.4	England and Wales (1988–90) 225.5
Denmark 273.9	Netherlands (1989–92) 225.0
Japan, Osaka 272.8	Switzerland, Vaud 224.2
England and Wales (1988–90) 261.1	Germany, Saarland 219.2
Singapore: Chinese 258.0	Norway 217.2
Norway 255.8	Finland (1987–92) 204.1
Finland (1987–92) 251.0	Singapore: Chinese 194.6
Sweden 240.7	Japan, Osaka 154.8
Spain, Zaragoza (1986–90) 238.8	Spain, Zaragoza (1986–90) 143.9

Source: Parkin et al 1997.[3]

occupational medicine. Subsequently, many other occupations are known to be associated with bladder cancer (Box 1.1).

Box 1.1 Chemicals, groups of chemicals, or industrial processes carcinogenic to humans

Aluminium production

Auramine manufacture

Boot and shoe manufacture and repair (certain occupations)

Coal gas production

Coal-tar pitches

Coke production

Furniture manufacture

Iron and steel founding

Isopropyl alcohol manufacture (strong-acid process)

Manufacture of magenta

Nickel refining

Rubber industry (certain occupations)

Underground hematite mining (with exposure to radon)

The continued search for environmental causes of cancer

The 20th century witnessed a continuous search for avoidable causes of cancer.

The powerful effects of tobacco smoke were quantified, and the debate still continues as to the effect of passive smoking.[6] Racial differences in incidence were observed.[7]

The discovery of hormones and the synthesis of artificial hormones led to observations on the effects of the two main sex hormones, oestrogen and testosterone, on various cancers.

The latter part of the 20th century led to an explosion of theories regarding the role of diet in cancer. Various diets have been devised, and the effect of adding compounds such as retinoids and carotenoids,[8] and vitamin C to an adequate diet continues to be discussed.[9]

Selenium, which is an essential trace element found in plants, enters the food chain by plant ingestion and is essentially dependent on soil concentration. Selenium may protect against the action of certain carcinogens.[10]

Almost all dietary chemicals are excreted through the urine after, in some cases, a chemical change in the liver. This mechanism presents carcinogens to the bladder lining. The preferred sites of cancer in the bladder are close to the ureteric orifices and to the trigone and bladder base where chemicals would be expected to linger longest. Metabolites of tar certainly find their way into the urine and, hence, to these sites. We are all exposed to synthetic chemicals if we think about it – gardening, hair dyeing, car repairs, preparing chemotherapy for patients, etc.

Surfaces of fruit may be coated with pesticides and water may have trace contamination.[11,12]

Even if we do not initially ingest these chemicals, if we smoke without washing our hands, traces are burned and find their way into the lungs, the bloodstream and finally the liver and bladder.[13]

Environmental exposure continues to be important.

The role of environmental agents continues to be debated[14,15] and it is likely to play as great a role in urological cancers for many years to come.

There is a wealth of publications about environmental agents in urological cancer and a Further Reading section follows the references.

REFERENCES

1. Dubos RJ. Man, medicine and environment. New York: Frederick A Praeger, 1968, p 94
2. Harras A. Cancer. Rates and risks, 4th edn. Washington: National Institute of Health, 1996
3. Parkin DM, Whelan SL, Ferlay J, Raymond L, Young J (eds) Cancer incidence in five continents, Vol. VII. IARC Scientific Publications No. 143. Lyon: International Agency for Research on Cancer, 1997
4. Pott P. Chirurgical observations relative to the cataract, the polypus of the nose, the cancer of the scrotum, *etc*. London: L Hawes, W Clarke and R Collins, 1775

5. Rehn L. Blasengeschwulste bei Fuchsin-Arbeitern. Arch Klin Chir 1895; 50:588–600
6. Peto J, Doll R. Passive smoking. Br J Cancer 1986; 54:381–383
7. Ross RK, Bernstein L, Lobo RA, et al. 5-alpha-reductase activity among Japanese and U.S. white and black males. Lancet 1992; 339:887–889
8. Ziegler RG. A review of epidemiologic evidence that carotenoids reduce the risk of cancer. J Nutr 1989; 119:116–122
9. Block G, Patterson B, Subar A. Fruit, vegetables and cancer prevention: a review of the epidemiologic evidence. Nutr Cancer 1992; 18:1–29
10. Giovannucci E. Selenium and risk of prostate cancer. Lancet 1998; 352:755–756
11. Blair A, Axelson O, Franklin C, et al. Carcinogenic effects of pesticides. In: The effect of pesticides on human health, Baker SR, Wilkinson CF (eds). Adv Modern Environ Toxicol, Princeton Scient. Publ., 1990, 8:201–260
12. Block G. Vitamin C and cancer prevention: the epidemiologic evidence. Am J Clin Nutr 1991; 53:270S–282S
13. Blair A, Zahm SH, Pearce NE, et al. Clues to cancer etiology from studies of farmers. Scand J Work Environ Health 1992; 18:209–215
14. Brennan P, Bogillot O, Cordier S, et al. Cigarette smoking and risk of bladder cancer in men: a pooled analysis of 11 case-control studies. Int J Cancer 2000; 86:289–294
15. Doll R, Peto R. The causes of cancer: quantitative estimates of avoidable risks of cancer in the United States today. J Natl Cancer Inst 1981; 1191–1308

FURTHER READING: POTENTIAL ASSOCIATIONS WITH CAUSATIVE AGENTS

Prostate

Barrett-Conner E, Garland C, McPhillips JB, et al. A prospective, population-based study of androstenedione, estrogens, and prostatic cancer. Cancer Res 1990; 50:169–173
Bosland M. The etiopathogenesis of prostate cancer with special reference to environmental factors. Adv Cancer Res 1988; 128:796–805
Graham S, Haughey B, Marshall J, et al. Diet in the epidemiology of carcinoma of the prostate gland. J Natl Cancer Inst 1983; 70:687–692
Honda GD, Bernstein L, Ross RK, et al. Vasectomy, cigarette smoking, and age at first sexual intercourse as risk factors for prostate cancer in middle-aged men. Br J Cancer 1988; 57:326–331
Kolonel LN, Yoshizawa CN, Hankin JH. Diet and prostatic cancer: a case-controlled study in Hawaii. Am J Epidemiol 1988; 127:999–1012
Nomura A, Heilbrun LK, Stemmermann GN, et al. Prediagnostic serum hormones and the risk of prostate cancer. Cancer Res 1988; 48:3515–3517
Ross RK, Shimizu H, Paganini-Hill A, et al. Case-control studies of prostate cancer in blacks and whites in Southern California. J Natl Cancer Inst 1987; 78:869–874

Testicular cancer

Brown LM, Pottern LM. Testicular cancer and farming. Lancet 1984; 1:1356
Brown LM, Pottern LM, Hoover RN. Prenatal and perinatal risk factors for testicular cancer. Cancer Res 1986; 46:4812–4816
Brown LM, Pottern LM, Hoover RN. Testicular cancer in young men: the search for causes of the epidemic increase in the United States. J Epidemiol Commun Health 1987; 41:349–354
Coldman AJ, Elwood JM, Gallagher RP. Sports activities and risk of testicular cancer. Br J Cancer 1982; 46:749–756
Depue RH, Pike MC, Henderson BE. Estrogen exposure during gestation and risk for testicular cancer. J Natl Cancer Inst 1983; 71:1151–1155
Karagas MR, Weiss NS, Strader CH, et al. Elevated intrascrotal temperature and the incidence of testicular cancer in noncryptorchid men. Am J Epidemiol 1989; 129:1104–1109
Mills PK, Newell GR, Johnston DE. Testicular cancer associated with employment in agriculture and oil and natural gas extraction. Lancet 1984; 1:207–210
Moss AR, Osmond D, Bacchetti P, et al. Hormonal risk factors in testicular cancer – a case-controlled study. Am J Epidemiol 1986; 124:39–52
Pottern LM, Brown LM, Hoover RN, et al. Testicular cancer risk among young men: role of cryptorchidism and inguinal hernia. J Natl Cancer Inst 1985; 74:377–381
Strader CH, Weiss NS, Daling JR. Vasectomy and the incidence of testicular cancer. Am J Epidemiol 1988; 128:56–63
Swerdlow AJ, Huttly SRA, Smith PG. Testicular cancer and antecedent diseases. Br J Cancer 1987; 55:97–103

Swerdlow AJ, Huttly SRA, Smith PG. Is the incidence of testis cancer related to trauma or temperature? Br J Urol 1988; 61:518–521

Tollerud DJ, Blattner WA, Fraser MC, et al. Familial testicular cancer and urogenital developmental anomalies. Cancer 1985; 55:1849–1854

Transitional cell cancer

Cantor KP, Hoover R, Hartge P, et al. Bladder cancer, drinking water source, and tap water consumption: a case-control study. J Natl Cancer Inst 1987; 79:1269–1279

Case RAM, Hosker ME, McDonald DB, et al. Tumours of the urinary bladder in the workmen engaged in the manufacture and use of certain dyestuff intermediates in the British Chemical Industry. Br J Ind Med 1954; 11:75–104

Hoover RN, Strasser PH, Child M, et al. Artificial sweeteners and cancer of the lower urinary tract. N Engl J Med 1980; 1:837–840

McLaughlin JK, Blot WJ, Mandel JS, et al. Etiology of cancer of the renal pelvis. J Natl Cancer Inst 1983; 71:287–291

Renal cancer

McLaughlin JK, Mandel JS, Blot WJ, et al. A population-based case-control study of renal cell carcinoma. J Natl Cancer Inst 1984; 72:275–284

McLaughlin JK, Blot WJ, Mehl ES, et al. Relation of analgesic use to renal cancer: population-based findings. J Natl Cancer Inst Monogr 1985; 69:217–222

McLaughlin JK, Blot WJ, Fraumeni JF Jr. Diuretics and renal cell cancer. J Natl Cancer Inst 1988; 80:378

McLaughlin JK, Silverman DT, Hsing AW, et al. Cigarette smoking and cancers of the renal pelvis and ureter. Cancer Res 1992; 52:254–257

Maclure M, Willett W. A case-controlled study of diet and risk of renal adenocarcinoma. Epidemiology 1990; 1:430–440

Yu MC, Mack TM, Hanisch R, et al. Cigarette smoking, obesity, diuretic use, and coffee consumption as risk factors for renal cell carcinoma. J Natl Cancer Inst 1986; 77:351–353

2

The nature of cancer

The case of M. Parent leads to the admission of cancer metastases: here a spontaneous eruption is succeeded by an identical eruption at another site
Joseph-Claude – Anthelme Recamier[1]

The survival of complex organisms depends on a staggeringly fast turnover of its constituent units. Only under exceptional circumstances does Nature favour repair: anything remotely shop-soiled or outworn is discarded and replaced. Theoretically this extravagance could be controlled from the production end, the rate of disposal of old cells being governed by the rate of production of new ones. For reasons unknown this is not what happens. In reality it is the rate of wastage that determines the rate of replacement. This implies a 'self-destruct' programme built into every cell and a sensitive feedback.[2]
TL Dormandy[2]

Over a lifetime, an individual has grown from a single-celled organism, to one with many millions of millions of cells. From this initial stem cell, tissues of a wide variety and complexity have been derived. In most cases, this growth process proceeds without incident and must have complex regulatory mechanisms to police cell growth and to keep the cells in order. Occasionally, developmental problems can occur, when the cells fail to fuse, e.g. hypospadias. Perhaps the greatest surprise of all is that this mechanism rarely fails in adulthood. The incidence of cancer rises with age and this is in part due to the number of cell divisions which have taken place and the possibility of error in cell divisions as well as a potential breakdown of repair mechanisms and senescence of the immune system.

BENIGN TUMOURS

There are occasions when tumours develop, when a cell starts growing and multiplying outside the normal regulatory pathways and can in theory expand indefinitely. A mass of cells may develop, which is in no way helpful to the body. However, most of these tumours are not a threat to the whole organism, because they remain localised and are not normally life threatening, unless they give rise to problems, e.g. due to pressure on vital structures or elaboration of excess normal products or harmful abnormal products. These benign tumours may function as though they were entirely normal tissues. The connections of surface molecules retain the tumour in one colony and the tumour remains localised. They may even have a fibrous capsule delineating the extent of the tumour.

DYSPLASIA

In most epithelial surfaces, new cells are developed in the basal layer and then the cells gradually move toward the surface.

In dysplasia, the dividing cells are not found solely in the basal layer, but are found scattered through the superficial layers of epithelium. This effect is seen specifically in cervical smears. Dysplastic areas may regress or may progress to carcinoma *in situ*. This is a much more severe form of dysplasia, where cell division and differentiation are more severely affected. The cells are undifferentiated and extremely variable in size. At this stage, however, the cells are above the basal lamina. If the cells transgress the basal lamina, then the specimen has become fully malignant.

MALIGNANT TUMOURS

Malignant tumours have a tendency to spread: they move from their local position and invade the surrounding tissues and set up separate colonies remote from the site of the primary growth. This second propensity is called metastasis.

Metastases are secondary tumours, remote from the primary tumour and which have spread through the bloodstream to a new location. Malignant tumours have two hallmarks:

*   invasion
*   metastasis.

These malignant cells are generally less well differentiated, as indeed they appear microscopically and their initial function may well have been lost, e.g. forming an impervious layer in the bladder, as transitional cells. The structure of a transitional cell is lost when it becomes malignant.

As the cells become more and more disorganised, the more malignant the tissue becomes, and many of the regulatory mechanisms appear to be lost, with the number of cell divisions.

Tumour cells have an alteration in normal cell-to-cell interactions and begin to lack the normal control of cell growth.

CELL–CELL RECOGNITION

Surface glycoproteins are important in cell recognition processes, with specific oligosaccharide chains allowing cells to recognise each other. Examples are:

*   ABO blood groups.
*   Major histocompatibility complex (MHC) antigens.

Adhesion molecules

There are four major families of cell adhesion molecules:

*   cadherins
*   immunoglobulin superfamily
*   selectins
*   integrins.

Cell adhesion molecules can be studied in the laboratory, using cell lines. A number of cell lines have lost the ability to cease division and have become immortal. Benign cells will only undergo a certain number of divisions, about 20, until they start to die off, but when a cell becomes immortalised, it carries on growing indefinitely in culture, as long as the appropriate nutrients are supplied.

Changes in immortalised cells in culture
In cell culture, many changes can occur: e.g.

*   there may be alterations in growth parameters of the cell
*   the requirement for growth factor may be reduced
*   there may be a loss of capacity for growth arrest.

Normally, when the concentrations of certain growth factors fall below a certain concentration, the cells become switched off as regards their growth. Transformed cells are unable to stop their growth and continue dividing.

Cells may also lose their need for anchorage and have lost their requirement for adherence. The cell may change its shape and its method of growth and also lose its contact inhibition of movement. Normally, cells will stop moving when they meet another cell, but this characteristic seems to get lost.

Potential reasons for observed changes
*   There is an increased mobility of surface proteins
*   Increased glucose transport
*   Reduced or absence of surface fibronectin
*   Changes in cytoskeleton, due to loss of actin microfilaments.

The cells may release transforming growth factors and may also elaborate protease, which digest proteins and allow erosion of the normal body tissue. An example of this is plasminogen activator, which cleaves the peptide bond in serum protein plasminogen, converting it to the protease plasmin.

There may be altered gene transcription, by over-expression, loss (by deletion) or mutation. This may lead to increased concentration of mRNAs which can now be measured.

Hormones

A hormone is a molecule produced by an endocrine cell that is released into the bloodstream and acts on specific receptors. Steroid hormones are synthesised from cholesterol and are hydrophobic.

The three mechanisms of cell signalling by hormones to surface receptors are:

- endocrine – cell to distant cell remote signalling using hormones
- paracrine – local cell to cell signalling
- autocrine – cells signalling back to themselves.

Cell surface receptors

Cell surface receptors are specific proteins that bind a signalling molecule and convert this binding into intracellular signals which alter the cell's behaviour.

Steroid receptors

Steroid receptors are not membrane-bound receptors, but soluble cytoplasmic proteins. Steroid receptors bind water-insoluble steroid, retinoid and thyroid hormones which pass through the lipid membrane.

Second messengers – how the message is relayed within the cell

The second messenger system is a set of intracellular molecules that is activated by cell surface receptors and affects cell function, producing a physiological response: e.g. AMP, GMP.

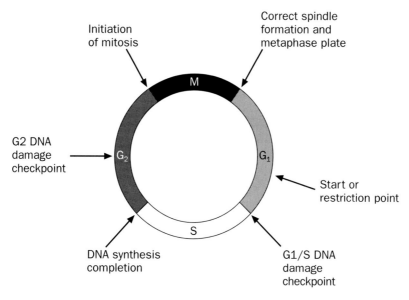

Figure 2.1 The cell cycle.

THE CELL CYCLE

Cells have a cycle of activity and inactivity (Figure 2.1):

- G1 – gap 1 – checkpoints occur at middle to end of this phase
- S – DNA synthesis
- G2 – gap 2 – checkpoint occurs
- M – mitosis cell division – the shortest phase.

Cyclins

Cyclins are proteins which are synthesised and then reabsorbed rapidly in phase with the phases of the cell cycle. Cyclins are named because of their cyclic accumulation and disappearance throughout the cell cycle.

Cyclins control the cell cycle by interacting with cyclin-dependent kinases (CDKs). These, in turn, are activated and stimulate cell cycle progression by phosphorylation of specific targets in the cell.

Cyclins C, D and E reach peak levels during the G1 phase and cyclins A and B1 reach peak levels during the S and G2 phases.[3]

Regulation of the cell cycle

The cell cycle is controlled by gene products which govern the transition from one phase to another. The intracellular concentrations of these products vary throughout the cell cycle.

S-phase protein and other factors

S-phase protein controls the transition from the G1 into the S phase:

- growth factors
- hormones
- mitogens (factors that induce mitosis).

THE CENTRAL DOGMA OF MOLECULAR BIOLOGY

The genetic material of the cell is deoxyribonucleic acid (DNA), which codes for the primary structures or amino acid sequence of the thousands of cellular proteins. DNA is found almost exclusively in the cell nucleus of human cells, although some is found in mitochondria. Mitochondrial DNA is inherited exclusively from the female line. DNA is the crown jewel of the cell and, as with crown jewels, does not move out of its protective nucleus but sends an intermediate molecule (mRNA or messenger ribonucleic acid), which is copied in a process called transcription. The RNA code is then translated into an amino acid sequence by a process which requires tRNA transfer and protein RNA structures called ribosomes.

What is a gene?

A gene is a linear sequence of nucleotides within the DNA which determines the linear sequence of amino acids in a polypeptide. Proteins may be composed of two or more polypeptide subunits which combine to form protein; the polypeptide subunits may be coded for by different genes. The human genome contains around 30,000 genes.

Only 0.1% of genome sequences are different between races, and these small differences account for genetic diversity, different response to medications, toxins and the environment.

In 1977, Sanger and his colleagues developed a method for sequencing the order of bases in DNA. Over 2,700,000 bases of draft human genome sequences are available in public databases and over a million are fully sequenced with an accuracy of 99.9%. Sequencing has allowed comparison of the genetic and physical distances along each chromosome. Genetic distance is measured in centimorgans (cM). The frequency of recombination which occurs at meiosis during the formation of spermatocytes or oocytes allows calculation of genetic distance.

The total haploid (i.e. unpaired) amount of DNA in organisms varies greatly – about 10^6 base pairs (bp) for mycoplasma, up to 10^{11} bp for some amphibians.

The human genome has 3×10^9 bp, equivalent to 0.9 metres of DNA double helix. Only about 10% of mammalian DNA is believed to code for protein.

Human genes can be transfected into animals and the single gene function either augmented or knocked out (gene knockout).

STRUCTURE OF DNA

DNA is a double helix consisting of two complementary antiparallel polynucleotide strands. Genetic information is stored along the length of the DNA and there are about 2 metres in every human cell. The molecular structure was discovered in 1953 by Watson and Crick. The order of bases in the nucleotides stores the genetic information.

DNA has a double helix and the two polynucleotide chains are coiled around a common axis, with the sugar phosphate backbone of each strand on the outside of the helix and the purine and pyrimidine bases projecting inwards, perpendicular to the axis of the helix. The two chains have opposite polarity, in that they are anti-parallel, one running from the 5' (5-prime) to the 3' end and the other from the 3' to the 5' end. The two strands are held together by hydrogen bonding between pairs of bases. Each nucleotide comprises a phosphate group, linked to a pentose sugar (deoxyribose), which is linked to either a purine or pyrimidine base: these are flat molecules containing nitrogen. The purine bases in DNA are adenine (A) and guanine (G). The pyrimidine bases are thymine (T) and cytosine (C). Guanine always pairs with cytosine (i.e. G–C) and adenine always pairs with thymine (i.e. A–T), a process called complementary base pairing.

Purine–pyrimidine
A–T
G–C

The nucleotides are linked together by a backbone of alternating pentose residues and phosphate groups, with the 5' carbon atom of one pentose ring connected to the 3' carbon atom of the adjacent pentose by a phosphate group, forming a 5'–3' phosphodiester linkage. Nucleic acids possess polarity in that at one end the terminal pentose bears the phosphate group, attached to its 5' carbon atom (referred to as the 5' end), whereas the other terminal pentose bears a free 3' hydroxyl group (referred to as the 3' end). At intervals, the DNA is wrapped around histone proteins and this forms a nucleosome.

It is a convention to write nucleic acid sequences with the 5' end on the left and they are often not specified.

Nuclear DNA is packaged into chromosomes: DNA plus proteins forms chromatin. Pairs of chromosomes are only visible at cell division, and in between only chromatin can be distinguished. The human chromosome complement or karyotype consists of two copies of the genome in 22 pairs of autosomes plus X and Y chromosomes. Chromosomes can be rearranged by loss, gain or breakage in diseased tissue.[3]

DNA REPLICATION

At cell division by mitosis the cells receive a diploid number of chromosomes. When germ cells are produced, at meiosis, each daughter cell receives only half of the total normal number of chromosomes, and is said to be haploid. Both strands of DNA contain complementary sequences of nucleotides, and therefore each strand can act as a template for a new strand. When DNA replication takes place, two complete double helices are produced from the original DNA, and each new DNA helix is identical to the original DNA double helix.

The two DNA strands are bound together by a large number of hydrogen bonds which are very difficult to disrupt. For replication to occur, the strands must be opened. In humans, DNA replication takes place in numerous places, allowing the cell to replicate quickly. When the replicating DNA is examined under an electron microscope, it is possible to see Y-shaped junctions in the DNA called replication forks. Any replication occurs in both directions and the forks move quickly at a rate of 100 nucleotide pairs per second in humans. The enzyme which accomplishes this is called DNA polymerase. DNA polymerase is so accurate that it makes only about one error in every 10^7 nucleotide pairs replicated. DNA polymerase has an error-correcting activity called proof-reading. It checks to make sure that the previous nucleotide added is correctly based-paired to the template: if it is correctly paired, the DNA polymerase removes the mispaired nucleotide and tries again.

When DNA is replicated during cell division, each of the strands of the parent DNA molecule act as a template for the synthesis of a new complementary strand, resulting in two daughter molecules, identical in sequence to the original. In each new molecule, therefore, one strand is derived from the parent DNA and the other is merely synthesised. Because the order of bases is programmed by the base pair rules, there should be complete fidelity in the DNA sequence and therefore a conservation of the genetic information.

DNA replication starts off by annealing of a short piece of primer RNA to the template. The 3′ OH group of this primer RNA tract is incorporated in the first base of the new DNA strand. This is then repeated until the parent strand is fully copied. The DNA is unwound, as the replication fork progresses. It can only go in one direction (5′ to 3′) and there is therefore one continuous leading strand and many discontinuous lagging strands, which are also called Okazaki fragments. An enzyme called DNA ligase later joins these Okasaki fragments. The RNA primers are then removed.

As a DNA molecule replicates, its two strands are pulled apart to form one or more Y-shaped replication forks. The enzyme DNA polymerase, which is situated in the fork, lays down a new complementary DNA strand on each parental strand, making two new double helical molecules. DNA polymerase replicates a DNA template, with less than one error in every 10^7 bases read. This is because the enzyme removes its own polymerisation errors as it moves along the DNA.

DNA polymerase can only work in one direction and so therefore the leading strand is replicated in a continuous fashion. On the lagging DNA strand, the DNA is synthesised by the polymerase in a discontinuous process, which could be considered as back stitching, making short fragments of DNA that are later joined up by the enzyme DNA ligase to make a single continuous DNA strand.[3]

INTRONS AND EXONS

The sequence of bases which code for a gene usually divide into coding regions called exons and non-coding regions are called introns. DNA is transcribed by the production of a single-stranded ribonucleic acid (RNA) molecule using one of the DNA strands as a template. This messenger RNA is processed to remove the non-coding regions and to modify each end. It then migrates into the cytoplasm, coming out of the nucleus; this is known as translation. It then meets up with ribosomes in the cytoplasm and a series of molecules known as transfer RNA (tRNA). Transfer RNA is usually associated with a specific amino acid. Each transfer RNA carries a three-base coding region, which corresponds to the three bases on the messenger RNA: the sequence of three bases is known as a codon and is specific for each amino acid.[3]

Reading the code

The nucleotides are read in groups of three. Each trio of nucleotides or triplet is called a codon, which codes for the incorporation of one amino acid into a polypeptide. There are 4^3 possibilities, i.e. 64 possible combinations. Each amino acid is coded for by more than one codon and the genetic code is therefore said to be degenerate. The genetic code is universal to all organisms, with the exception of mitochondrial DNA, where a number of variant codon segments exist. Three of the 64 triplets (UAA, UAG and UGA) do not code for amino acids; they specify the terminal of polypeptide chain synthesis and are known as stop codons. Translation of the polypeptide starts at the codon AUG, which also codes for internal methionine residues. Hence, all newly synthesised polypeptide chains start with methionine.

Near the start site of the gene is a site at which RNA polymerase binds. This is frequently the sequence TATA and is known as a TATA box.[3]

Messenger RNA

Messenger RNA is different from DNA in that it has ribose rather than deoxyribose as its pentose sugar and also it uses the pyrimidine base uracil (U instead of thymine, T):

In mRNA: U always pairs with A

There is normally more than one ribosome on a mRNA chain during protein synthesis and this collection of ribosomes, visible with an electron microscope, is termed a polysome.

Post-translational modification of protein

Post-translational modification of proteins is crucial to protein function. Proteins are modified after the polypeptide chain is formed by various chemical processes and the chain is folded and formed into its secondary and tertiary forms. In some instances, other proteins called chaperones associate with the protein at certain stages of folding to prevent incorrect liaisons being formed. The protein is led into the endoplasmic reticulum by signal peptides, some of which are made in the Golgi apparatus.

Error avoidance and correction in replication

The DNA preliminaries are incapable of starting a new DNA chain, because of the proofreading feature. DNA synthesis is primed by an RNA preliminary called primase, which makes RNA. These are called primers and are subsequently erased and replaced with DNA. DNA repair enzymes continually scan the DNA and correct replication mistakes and replace damaged nucleotides. This is made particularly easy because of the complementary nature of the DNA, using the other strand as a template.

Lesions in the DNA occur in both replication and transcription: these may terminate any further replication and can be termed lethal. Any errors which creep in are dealt with by mismatched repair protein, which monitors the newly replicated DNA and repairs copying mistakes. DNA damage caused by chemical reaction to ultraviolet irradiation is repaired by a variety of enzymes that recognise damaged DNA and excise a short stretch of the DNA strand, with the error. The missing DNA is resynthesised by repair DNA and uses the undamaged strand as a template. DNA ligase reseals the DNA to complete the repair process.

DNA DAMAGE BY OTHER AGENTS

Damage may be fatal for the cell or produce mutation, i.e. non-lethal damage but damaging cell progeny. Mutations may be generated, and other forms of damage include oxidative damage by superoxide and hydroxide radicals, and alkylation induced by electrophilic alkylating agents. Bulky adducts, which are large bulky chemicals such as pyrimidine dimers, distort the double helix and cause localised denaturation.

Agents that cause DNA damage include:

- X-rays
- ultraviolet light: produces distortion, which promotes chemical cross-linking between two adjacent thymine residues, producing distortion
- chemical mutagens: base analogues; chemical modifiers; and intercalators.

Mutagenesis

Physical mutagens, such as ionising radiation in the form of X-rays or ultraviolet light, cause the target molecules to lose electrons. These electrons then cause chemical alterations to DNA in the form of strand breakage, base destruction and sugar destruction. Base analogues can cause direct mutagenesis. Nitrose acid deaminates cytosine to produce uracil. Alkylating agents produce chemical changes which interfere with transcription and replication. These chemical mutagens are often termed carcinogens, since they cause cancer.

The Ames test

The Ames test is performed in Salmonella to test for mutagenicity. It is an effective mechanism for predicting the carcinogenic potential of a compound, since the mechanisms are essentially the same in all organisms. It is an assay which measures the ability of the mutagen to cause mutations in the Salmonella, which should be proportional to its ability to cause mutation. The presence of a liver extract modifies the mutagen, activating it in the way that it would be activated by passage through the liver.

Cancer-causing viruses

Both DNA and RNA viruses can cause cancer, but they do this by different mechanisms. DNA viruses carry foreign genes, which can cancel out the normal cellular control mechanisms. RNA viruses often carry mutated copies of normal cellular genes, as well as their own reverse transcriptase, which they require for their replication. Both DNA and RNA viruses can cause tumours by insertion in or near a proto-oncogene.

Nearly every step in cellular signalling and regulation systems has provided examples of proto-oncogenes:

- hormones
- tyrosine
- kinase receptors (*erb*-B)
- signal transduction (*ras*)
- DNA-binding protein (*erb*-A nuclear receptor).

Various methods of identification of oncogenes have been used, including analyses of sequences near the site of viral insertion, the investigation of chromosomal translocations, the sequence of tumour causing viruses and the tranfection of cells with DNA from tumours.

Alterations, which cause proto-oncogenes to become activated to oncogenes, include point mutations outside of the coding region. Changes in the level of activity of the protein include mutations in the protein, which change its activity, and mutations or amplification, which changes the total amount of protein being expressed in the cell.

The development of tumours is thought to require multiple mutations, and other independent mutations may be required.

Oncogenes

It is known that certain genes in an individual can elaborate a protein which can transform cells in culture or induce cancer in neighbouring normal cells by giving the cells a growth advantage and allowing unregulated growth (Table 2.1).

Table 2.1 Difference between oncogenes and tumour suppressor genes[5]	
Oncogene	**Tumour suppressor gene**
Gene active in tumour	Gene inactive in tumour
Specific translocations/point mutations	Deletions or mutations
Mutations rarely hereditary	Mutations can be inherited
Dominant at cell level	Recessive at cell level
Broad tissue specificity	Considerable tumour specificity
Especially leukaemia and lymphoma	Solid tumours

Many oncogenes are known: some are cellular genes called proto-oncogenes which, when altered, become oncogenes. Oncogenes produce oncoproteins, which can transform certain cells, turning them from benign to malignant cells. This mechanism is an example of a single-hit mechanism or abnormality – one abnormality is sufficient to trigger the mechanism.

It is worth remembering that the proto-oncogene is spelt with a 3-letter lower case characterisation and italicised, but the protein product is given a capital letter and is not italicised.

Oncogenes were initially identified in viruses and tumour cell DNA. The *ras* genes are common oncogenes which are found in both animal and human tumours.

Proteins controlling cell growth
There are a number of proteins which control cell growth, e.g. growth factors, growth factor receptors, intracellular signal transducers, nuclear transcription factors and cell-cycle control proteins. Genes for these proteins can produce oncogenes.

Proto-oncogenes
Proto-oncogenes are normal genes which can change into oncogenes, e.g. the proto-oncogene *bcl*-2 prevents cells from dying and is used in memory cells in the immune system. If activated inappropriately, white cells can become leukaemic or lymphomatous.

Proto-oncogene to oncogene
Oncogene activation from proto-oncogenes leads to abnormal cell control. Activation of oncogenes occurs by:

- translocation
- amplification
- point mutation in an oncogene.

Tumour suppressor genes

Tumour suppressor genes, also known as anti-oncogenes, normally inhibit tumorigenesis by a two-hit mechanism, as described by Knudson.[4] Both copies of the gene must be inactivated

(Table 2.1). This leads to loss of growth retardation or regulation, e.g. the *VHL* gene in clear cell renal cancer. This has been compared to a car losing its brakes.

p53
The p53 gene has been dubbed the guardian of the genome. Over 50% of human tumours contain mutations of this gene. All vertebrate species have a gene that encodes a protein called p53 (p = protein, 53 = molecular weight in kilodaltons or kDa). The p53 protein has a short half-life, being synthesised and degraded rapidly. Cellular damage causes p53 to be stabilised.

Roles of p53
Three major roles of p53 have been identified:
- pausing and repairing damage – transcription activator – regulating certain genes involved in cell division
- inhibiting cell division – as a G1 restriction point for DNA damage – if there has been excess DNA damage (e.g. ultraviolet damage)
- participating in the initiation of apoptosis.

Absence or alteration of p53
Absence or alteration of p53 allows cells to survive effects of mutation, and may permit cells to go into a persistent dividing state.

Other effects of absence or alteration include:

- cells may survive hypoxic conditions
- certain cancer viruses may be permitted to replicate
- cells with damaged DNA may continue dividing.

If a p53 gene abnormality is found in a biopsy, it may be a marker of poor prognosis.

Telomeres and telomerase

Normal cells die out in the course of 30–40 replications but cancer cells continue to divide. When normal cells divide, the end portion of the chromosome, called the telomere, is eroded. Cancer cells develop a repair mechanism to renew the telomeres and this may be a mechanism for targeting cancer cells.

Telomeres, which are composed of tandem repeated DNA sequences and their associated proteins, have multiple functions, including maintaining the integrity of chromosomes. Unless telomerase, an enzyme, is fully active, progressive telomere loss results with each cell division, as a result of the end replication problem.

Telomerase is a ribonuclear protein which is inactive from about 20 weeks of human development when the process of telomeric attrition is thought to begin. Immortal cancer cells solve this problem by upregulating telomerase activity and stabilising telomeres, and the inhibition of telomerase can reverse the immortal phenotype, causing death in some cancer cells.[6]

APOPTOSIS

Apoptosis is derived from the Greek for leaves falling off a tree. It is essentially programmed cell death and is a natural part of the cycle of growth. Apoptosis depends upon the activation of a terminal effector pathway; central in this pathway is a family of cysteine-containing aspartate-specific proteases called caspases. When these enzymes are activated and leave their substrates, the structural manifestations of apoptosis are seen, with characteristic alterations in the cytoskeleton, cell surface and nucleus.

Caspase activation is triggered by a variety of signals such as injury, affecting mitochondria, the cell membrane and chromatin. These damage-associated signals interact with physiological signalling pathways activated through surface receptors, notably members of the tumour necrosis factor (TNF) receptor family (TNFr1, TNFr2 and DR4). Any viral genes are surrogates for endogenous genes, coding death inhibitory molecules. Even lytic viruses possess apoptosis inhibitors and transforming viruses uniformly encode apoptosis inhibitory inhibitor genes. Apoptosis is activated by the tumour suppressor gene p53.

Most cytotoxic agents used in tumour therapy activate apoptosis. They may have other actions also of course.[7–9]

Cell adhesion molecules in cancer

Qualitative and quantitative changes in adhesion receptor expression have been found in a majority of human tumours, using experimental model systems and in-vivo immunolocalisation studies. There may be a decrease in cell-matrix adhesion or loss of intercellular adhesion. There is some evidence that adhesion receptors and their associated cytoskeletal proteins can transmit growth stimulatory and/or inhibitory intercellular signals.[10–12]

Matrix metalloproteinases in cancer

Tumour cell invasion is now regarded as an abnormally regulated form of physiological invasion. Physiological invasion occurs in angiogenesis, tissue morphogenesis and placental trophoblast implantation. These processes involve a specific set of fibrous protein degrading enzymes, and important representatives of these enzymes are the matrix metalloproteinases (MMPs), which are family of zinc-dependent proteases, which break down extracellular matrix proteins such as collagens, fibronectin and laminin. The enzyme activity of MMPs is regulated within the tissue by a family of endogenously produced inhibitors called tissue inhibitors of metalloproteinases (TIMPs). The balance between MMP and TIMP production is one factor in determining whether or not cell invasion occurs.

Some investigators believe that cancer may be viewed as a disease of the cell cycle and its control.[13]

Cytokines

Cytokines are soluble mediators of intercellular communication. They contribute to a chemical signalling system that regulates development, tissue repair, haemopoiesis, inflammation and the immune response. One cytokine can influence the production of response to many other cytokines. There are over 100 effector molecules. Cytokines influence communication between tumour and host cells. They may control the tumour microenvironment, providing the milieu for the tumour to grow and spread. They can produce growth factors, inflammatory cytokines and chemo-attractin cytokines called chemokines.

The production of lymphocyte-associated cytokines may trigger a specific immune response against a tumour.

Cytokine therapies have been used to increase the immune response to tumour cell antigens. They may act directly on the tumour, as well as on the stroma of the tumour. Cytokine treatments may regulate tumour cell proliferation, differentiation, survival, mortality and cell-to-cell and cell-to-matrix interactions. They may also influence host cell functions, such as neovascularisation, extracellular matrix synthesis, leucocyte infiltration, stromal cell proliferation and local immune response.

Interleukin 2 (IL2) has been successful in the treatment of renal cell carcinoma. Colony-stimulating factors may accelerate bone marrow recovery after myelotoxic therapies.

Growth factor receptors in human cancer

Growth factor receptors may function as soluble diffusible molecules or as cell surface anchor proteins. The growth factor receptors can be altered in cancer cells, leading to deregulation of growth and tumour formation. Overexpression or mutation of these receptors can lead to excessive growth stimulation.

Immunotherapy for cancer

Tumour-specific antigens were first shown in 1953. Transportation of tumours between genetically identical mice showed that recipient mice injected with tumour cells developed immune responses which protected against challenge from the same tumour cells.

Multi-drug resistance

Tumours can become refractory to the effects of chemotherapy. This may be termed multi-drug resistance. This is an acquired characteristic and can occur in renal cancer; it is distinct from intrinsic drug resistance. One type of multi-drug resistance is the result of amplification of a specific chromosomal component of a gene concerned with membrane transport (adenosine-triphosphatase or ATPase). ATPase is thought to export a broad range of drugs, and induction of this enzyme can amplify the effects and allow the cell to expel the chemotherapy drug with increasing efficiency and thus diminish the killing effect of the agent.

Tumour initiators and promoters

A tumour initiator, such as a mutagen, while being able to cause a tumour, can also create mutations in the DNA, which might be unmasked by exposure to a promoter at any time in the future.

A promoter may be any substance or factors, including wounding, which alters the expression of the cell and masks the effects of the initiator.

Angiogenesis in cancer

As tumours become larger, they depend on a dedicated blood supply. Initially, they are able to exist in an interstitial substance of the body and oxygen can only diffuse for a very short distance. Pro- and anti-angiogenic molecules can be produced from cancer cells, to promote angiogenesis. There are a number of molecules which promote vascular growth, such as vascular endothelial growth factor (VEGF) and angiopoietin.

TECHNIQUES IN MOLECULAR BIOLOGY

Immunohistochemistry

Protein expression in cells can be used to predict outcome and behaviour of cells, because there are a vast number of antibodies available commercially. Protein products such as tumour markers, products of tumour suppressive genes, oncogenes and tumour invasion molecules, cell-cycle regulatory proteins and targets of chemotherapy can be assessed.

This technique is used to localise p53 in tumours.

Because of the thrust to higher sensitivity, there are various methods being developed to amplify the original protein level, without sacrificing specificity.

Analysing gene structure
Southern blotting
Professor Ed Southern first described his method of analysing a gene structure to detect specific DNA sequences. The technique works essentially by hybridising DNA segments in solution to DNA segments fixed to a membrane.

The DNA fragments in the gel are denatured by soaking the gel in alkali. The fragments are transferred from the gel to an island membrane by a capillary transfer procedure, since the original fragments are too fragile. The membrane can then be incubated with a single-stranded label probe for the gene, which it has been tested for.

The bound probe is then detected by autoradiography or by immunodetection of non-radioactive probes.

Northern blotting
Northern blotting detects mRNA rather than genomic DNA. Northern blotting determines the size and amount of messenger RNA. The RNA is extracted and treated by electrophoresis on a gel. After electrophoresis the RNA is transferred to an island membrane and linked to the membrane by ultraviolet illumination. A labelled DNA or RNA probe is hybridised to the Northern blot.

Western blotting
Western blotting is used to detect specific proteins.

Comparison of blotting techniques
A comparison of blotting techniques is shown in Table 2.2.

Fluorescence in-situ hybridisation – FISH

This technique is used to hybridise probes to RNA within cells in tissue sections. The probes may be either radioactive or non-radioactive. Until recently, in-situ hybridisation was performed exclusively with radioactive probes. More recently, probes labelled with haptens such as biotin and other agents have allowed non-radioactive methods such as fluorescence to localise specific RNA within cells. This has led to savings in time and better reproducibility. These chromosome-specific probes can detect specific chromosome metaphase spreads or interface nuclei and can also detect an extra chromosome in aneuploid cells, tumour cells or hybrid cells. They attach to a target chromosome. This tech-

Table 2.2 Comparison of blotting techniques

Blot	Electrophoreses	Type of gel	Probe
Southern	DNA	Agarose	DNA
Northern	RNA	Agarose	RNA
Western	Protein	Polyacrylamide	Protein
South-western	Protein	Polyacrylamide	DNA

nique is used in mapping studies. Different probes can be used in the same experiment.[14]

The polymerase chain reaction (PCR)

This technique allows the production of large quantities of one specific region of DNA without cloning. It requires only small amounts of genomic DNA and specific DNA sequences can be amplified from single cells. It generates a large amount of specific DNA fragments from a complex genome. The process is based on a serious of cyclical enzymatic reactions. Both small and large areas can be amplified.

Many small fragments can be amplified by DOP, in a technique of amplification called DOP-PCR (DOP = degenerate oligonucleotide primed PCR). It results in amplification of many small fragments and gives a melange of DNA-amplified portions.

The template

Single-stranded molecules are produced from double-stranded DNA by melting the two strands apart at high temperature. The target sequence is then flanked on either side by oligonucleotide primers, The target sequence is therefore amplified. The original DNA polymerase was extracted from *Escherichia coli*, but now the use of thermophilic bacterium (*Thermus aquaticus*), which is not inactivated by the denaturation step, and thermal cyclers can rapidly change temperature at preset intervals. This technique has revolutionised DNA study.

THE IMMUNE SYSTEM

For the same man was never attacked twice – never at least fatally.
Thucydides (460–400 BC) The History of the Peleponnesian War:[20] commenting on the plague of Athens

From the earliest time in his development, man may have been subject to depredations by foreign organisms. A number of natural immune mechanisms have developed to repel these organisms. The skin and mucous membranes have a specific barrier function, but microorganisms can penetrate these barriers. The fatty acids secreted by the skin repel many bacteria but, occasionally, microorganisms can enter the body. They are generally phagocytosed by white cells or polymorphonuclear leucocytes or larger scavenging cells called macrophages. Many microorganisms are broken down by these mechanisms, but some have produced mechanisms that enable them to survive, either by producing toxins which destroy phagocytes or by developing a particularly strong coat which resists breakdown, e.g. pneumococci.

The complement system is an important non-specific defence system; it can produce proteins which coat the microorganisms and allow increased efficiency of phagocytosis. This process is called opsonisation. Complement produces proteins which enliven the cell membranes of microorganisms. The attack of microorganisms can be intra- or extracellular. A range of white cells called natural killer (NK cells) act specifically against viruses and tumours.

As microorganisms evolved, the body had to evolve mechanisms to deal with the increasing complexity of their assaults. Humans evolved a system of adaptive immunity based on the lymphocyte, a cell found only in vertebrates. This allowed the preservation of immune memory, so that if the body has encountered a foreign assault before, it remembers the nature of the coating proteins and is able to mount a secondary response.

Lymphocytes are divided into two types:

* B lymphocytes – so-called because of their derivation from bone marrow. They give rise to an antibody-mediated immune response.
* T lymphocytes – they give rise to a cell-mediated (T) immune response.

T cells recognise both foreign antigens and also normal molecules found on the surface of cells which they meet.

Peripheral blood normally contains 79% of T

cells, 10% of B cells and approximately 10% of NK cells. T cells mount a response called the cytotoxic T-cell response which destroys viruses but can also lead to transplant rejection.

T cells have a further action in that they are able to modify the function of other non-specific cells and elaborate the production of soluble molecules known as cytokines.

T lymphocytes pass through the thymus before they become fully immunocompetent. B cells reach maturity in the bone marrow without issuing forth into the body.

Lysis of virally infected cells involves the recognition of viral antigens and the host cell by the T-cell receptor. This causes receptor aggregation and a redirection of the T-cells production apparatus towards the infected cell.

B lymphocytes

B lymphocytes make and secrete antibodies. When they encounter a foreign antigen, they go through several cycles of cell division and then differentiate into specialised antibody-secreting cells called plasma cells.

T lymphocytes

T-cell receptors for antigen were identified in 1993. The receptors consist of two protein chains, rather similar to chains of immunoglobulin. When T lymphocytes first encounter an antigen, they undergo clonal expansion. Each antigen-specific T cell may increase to produce a few hundred cells. The affinity of the T-cell receptor remains the same T-cell memory and therefore resides in increased numbers of the specific T cells. Functions of T lymphocytes are given in Table 2.3 and functions and properties of cytokines in Table 2.4.

Stem cells

The body is continually turning over cells, particularly in the haemopoietic system and in the lin-

---

Table 2.3 T-lymphocyte functions[5]

Function	Cells involved	
In vivo	CD4	CD8
Delayed-type hypersensitivity	++	+/−
Graft rejection	++	++
Tumour rejection	++	++
Graft versus host response	++	++
Protection against viral and fungal infection	++	++
Protection against bacterial infection	++	+
In vitro		
Help for antibody responses	++	−
Mixed lymphocyte responses – proliferation	++	+
Mixed lymphocyte responses – cytotoxicity	+/−	++
Proliferation to mitogens	++	++
Proliferation to soluble antigens	++	−
Cytotoxicity against specific antigens (in association with MHC[a])	+/−	++
Production of cytokines	++	+

[a]MHC = major histocompatibility complex.

Table 2.4 Functions and properties of cytokines[5]		
Cytokine	**Main effects**	**Molecular weight (Da) and other properties**
Cloned and characterised cytokines		
Interleukin-1α	Activation of T cells	17,500; produced by many cells
Interleukin-1β	Pyrogenic response	17,500; produced by many cells
Interleukin-2	Growth of T cells	13,500; from T and NK cells
Interleukin-3	Growth of haemopoietic stem cells	18,000–30,000; T cell product
Interleukin-4	Growth and differentiation of T and B cells	15,000–18,000; T cell product
Interleukin-5	Effects on B cells and granulocytes	20,000–22,000; T cell product
Interleukin-6	B-cell differentiation by many other effects also	21,000; produced by many cells
Interleukin-7	Growth of B cells	25,000
Interleukin-10	Inhibition of Th-1 cells	16,000–20,000; produced by Th2 cells
Interleukin-15	Growth of T cells	15,000; produced by many non-lymphoid cell types
Chemokines (e.g. interleukin-8)	Chemotaxis of lymphocytes, granulocytes and macrophages	8000; a large family of peptides, produced by many cell types
Interferon-α	Inhibition of viral replication	15,000; produced by many cells
Interferon-γ	Increase of major histocompatibility complex (MHC) expression; inhibition of viral replication	38,000; T cell product
Tumour necrosis factor-α	Necrosis of tumours, pyrogenic	25,000 and multimers
Tumour necrosis factor-β	Cytotoxic *in vitro*	25,000 and multimers
Leukaemia inhibitory factor	Inducer if myeloid differentiation	20,000; produced by many cells
Colony-stimulating factors	Promote growth and maturation of progenitor cells	Various

ings of the gastrointestinal (GI) tract and in the testicles. Production in the testicle is generally in a steady state, but where there are problems of GI erosion or bleeding, then there must be an upregulation of production. Mature cells are derived from more primitive cells and these are known as stem cells. These stem cells appear to have a totipotent ability to differentiate into different types of cells. Stem cells seem capable of sus-

tained self-renewal. There is considerable interest as to how stem cells persist in the body. They may populate the body during embryogenesis, to supply a lifetime need. The second hypothesis is that these stem cells can reproduce themselves, to produce daughter cells with similar potential. This second model means that as the stem cells are recruited: there is no reduction in the total number of stem cells.

Table 2.5 Historical overview of genetics (reproduced with permission from the American Urological Association Office of Education: Bova/Getzenberg/Brooks/Bookstein).[22]

Period	Development
Ancient Greek and Chinese civilisations	Semen + menstrual blood = babies
1677	Publication by Hartsoecker and others of drawings of tiny humanoid 'humunculi' in heads of sperm
1856–63	Mendel performs experiments that demonstrate the presence of discrete units responsible for the expression of individual characteristics
1869	Miescher found that nuclei contain material that is not a protein, carbohydrate, or fat; calls substance 'Nuclein'
1879	Flemming names easily stainable nuclear material chromatin
1902	Garrod recognises first human example of Mendel's patterns of inheritance in Alkaptonurics (homozygous recessive)
1928	Griffith lays foundation for discovery of DNA by showing that dead capsule forming pneumococci can transfer material allowing non-capsule forming bacteria to form capsules
1944	Avery, MacLeod, McCarty provide first proof that DNA is material of heredity by proving that naked DNA can achieve the results of Griffith's experiment. Highly controversial for several years
1951	Wilkins and Franklin produce X-ray diffraction pattern of DNA
1952	Wilkins and Chase put to rest doubts that DNA is genetic material
1955	Watson and Crick suggest double-helical structure of DNA and method of DNA replication (*Nature* April 25)
1956	Tjio and Levan: first correct report of number of human chromosomes – 46
1960s	Banding techniques for chromosomes (Giemsa, other) devised
1970	Arber, Nathans and Smith discover restriction enzymes
1970	Baltimore, Temin, Mitzutani describe reverse transcription of RNA to DNA
1972	Berg clones first genes – SV40 and lambda phage
1975	Southern describes method for detecting specific DNA sequences by 'hybridising' DNA segments in solution to DNA segments fixed to a membrane
1977	Maxam and Gilbert describe a method for DNA sequencing
1980	Amgen, one of the first biotech companies, formed
1981	McKusick first publishes *Mendelian inheritance in man*
1983	Mullis describes PCR
1984	Human Genome Project first steps
1985	Greider and Blackburn describe telomerase
1989	Erythropoeitin, first biotech drug, approved
2001	Human genome sequence published

GENOMICS

Genomics is the study of the entire genome, the proteins that are encoded and their control (Table 2.5). *Proteomics* is the study of the interactions of the proteins, which results from genomic expression.

Gene therapy

To understand how gene therapy is constructed, remember that DNA generates RNA, which generates protein: i.e.

DNA → RNA → Protein

This process comprises three basic steps:

1. replication, making DNA copies from DNA
2. transcription, making RNA from DNA
3. translation, making protein from RNA.

The first two steps occur in the nucleus in human cells. Translation occurs in the cytoplasm. In diseases where genes are implicated, it is first necessary to identify whether the defect is due to a single gene or to a complex number of genes. It is also worth knowing whether the disease is acquired or inherited.

Once the gene or genes are identified, the type of intervention strategy has to be developed. This usually involves gene replacement, often with accompanying modulator genes. The decision has to be taken whether general expression or targeted expression is used. Once the genes and their mechanism have been discovered, a vector must be selected. This can be either a viral vector or a non-viral vector, such as a liposome or occasionally naked DNA. Finally, the method of gene delivery has to be decided. The agent used to introduce the new or altered gene is called a vector.

Viral vectors

Various viruses can be used. The retrovirus integrates the gene and prevents stable expression: the retrovirus is mainly used *in vitro*, because it usually produces random gene integration and delivers genes into dividing cells only, and could, of course, be used to integrate foreign genes into cancer cells.

Adenoviruses have also been used and they have a large capacity for gene insertion, but a low efficiency of infection. Patients may be immune to the virus.

Poxviruses do not need dividing cells and have a large capacity for gene insertion, but individuals may be immune to the virus. The poxvirus does not enter the nucleus.

Dendritic cells

Dendritic cells are one of the most important members of the antigen-presenting cells. They have a critical part to play in primary antigen-dependent T-cell responses. The T cells become sensitised, and become capable of recognising tumour cells and occasionally lysing. Dendritic cells are found throughout the body, but are normally obtained from peripheral blood or bone marrow. Dendritic cells can be cultured from peripheral blood monocytes. They express high levels of Class I and Class II major histocompatibility complexes (MHC proteins). The dendritic cells can be presented with appropriate tumour antigens and it is possible to use subsequent preparations as dendritic cell-based vaccines.

Recommended courses on molecular and cell biology

Techniques and Applications of Molecular Biology
Department of Biological Sciences
University of Warwick
Coventry CV4 7AL
UK
Tel: Coventry (01203) 523540
The Cellular and Molecular Basis of Cancer: Imperial College School of Medicine, Hammersmith Hospital, London, UK.
Understanding Molecular Technology and its Application to Urology: American Urological Association.
Gene Manipulation in Medicine and Gene Therapy: American Urological Association.

STAGING OF TUMOURS

The more advanced the tumour is at detection, the more likely it is to kill the patient. To prepare different treatments, it is essential that the case mix in each group of treatments is comparable. The only way of ensuring that this is genuinely so, is to randomise patients. However, patients may be assessed on a case control basis, using historical controls.

In order to compare like with like, the concept of staging has evolved. To allow comparison of results between centres, the TNM staging has been produced: this stands for tumour, node and metastases. This has been produced by the UICC (International Union Against Cancer). The presence or absence of involved lymph nodes is indicated. If there are no metastases, the stage is M0, but M1 indicates the presence of metastases. MX indicates whether the information is unknown. These are the bones of a system, which is constantly being refined and updated and allows comparison of results between centres. It aids planning of therapy and, most importantly, indicates prognosis.

GENERAL NOTES ON THERAPIES OF CANCER

Radiotherapy

Radiotherapy is the practice of using ionising radiation to disrupt and execute tissues which are believed to be malignant. Different forms of radiation are used to produce ionisation of molecules within the tissues. The physics of the particles is well understood.

Radiation produces damage by striking electrons out of atoms, which causes their ionisation. As part of this process, free radicals are produced in the tissue: these agents then attack DNA, breaking the DNA strands. There are a number of DNA repair mechanisms, although it is only when both strands are broken that the cell dies.

The particles which cause the destruction
Most treatments use high-energy X-ray photons, generated nowadays in linear accelerators.

There has been an increasing escalation in the energies used to generate the X-ray beams. These energies are measured in either kilovolts (kV) or megavolts (MV). The penetrating ability of the photons is proportional to the energy, i.e. the greater the number of volts, the deeper the penetration.

Radioisotopes may be in the form of permanent implants or may be administered in the form of injections, such as strontium 89. Strontium is taken up preferentially by bone, where the tissues mistake the strontium for calcium.

There has been a great deal of effort made to measure the biological effect. Radiation response is believed to be a balance between repair, re-oxygenation, and re-assortment and re-population of cells. It has also been recognised that some cells are more sensitive to damage than others. Fractionation of radiation timing can be very important in achieving maximum cell kill. Cells may recover between 4 and 6 hours.

Chemotherapy

Antimetabolites
Antimetabolites, which interfere with normal metabolic agents, include:

- methotrexate, a folic acid antagonist
- pyrimidine antagonist – 5-fluorouracil (5-FU)
- purine antagonists, e.g. 6-mercaptopurine (6-MP) and 6-thioguanine (6-TG).

Antibiotics
Certain antibiotics have been found to have antitumour properties and include:

- anthracyclines, such as doxorubicin, mitoxantrone, dactinomycin
- mitomycin C, which is derived from streptomyces fungus, and inhibits DNA synthesis by both cross-linking and alkylating DNA.

Podophyllotoxins
These are derived from an American mandrake plant: examples include etoposide.

Miscellaneous agents

Procarbazine

This agent is a weak monoamine oxidase inhibitor, which inhibits the action of RNA and DNA.

Hydroxyurea

This agent blocks the action of ribonucleotide diphosphate reductase and inhibits DNA synthesis.

L-Asparaginase

This enzyme acts by removing asparagine from the circulation, depriving tumour cells, which are unable to make asparagine because they have no or only low levels of asparagine synthetase.

Alkyloids

These are plant extracts from the periwinkle and act as spindle poisons, e.g. vincristine and vinblastine.

Mechanisms of action of cytotoxic drugs

Alkylating agents

These drugs work by binding chemical moieties in proteins and nucleic acids. They comprise probably the largest group of cytotoxic drugs. Examples include cyclophosphamide, ifosfamide, cisplatin, melphalan, mustine, chlorambucil, thiotepa, BiCNU (carmustine) and cis-chlorethylnitrosourea (CCNU). When cyclophosphamide is used, mesna must be given concurrently to protect the bladder from the toxic metabolite acrolein.

Cisplatin

Cisplatin has a half-life of about 40 min. It is excreted through the kidneys. Creatinine clearance is normally measured before treatment. The patient must be well hydrated prior to treatment and it is important that a good diuresis is maintained during the 24 hours following administration. Cisplatin has significant toxicity, which includes renal impairment, neuropathy, high tone hearing loss, and short-term GI toxicity. Cisplatin must be protected from light.

Carboplatin

Carboplatin is an analogue of cisplatin that has less renal toxicity and causes much less nausea and vomiting. Although having significantly less toxicity to the kidneys, and having no neurotoxicity or ototoxicity, carboplatin has been shown to be inferior in comparative studies to cisplatin and no further trials are recommended. It has a small place where cisplatin cannot be used.

LANDMARKS IN UNDERSTANDING OF CANCER

Landmarks are shown in Table 2.6.

Period	Achievement
	Table 2.6 Landmarks in understanding cancer
1655	Robert Hooke uses an early microscope to identify cells as individual units of life
1663–1750	Claude Gendron recognises cancer as arising locally and that its removal can be curative
1753	James Lind treats scurvy and uses first controlled trial
1775	Percivall Pott associates environment with scrotal cancer in chimney sweeps
1838	Johannes Muller describes abnormalities of cancer cells
1866	Gregor Mendel promulgates his findings on heredity
1889	Schinzinger proposes relationship between ovarian function and breast cancer
1894–96	Beatson describes palliation of breast cancer by ovariectomy. Rann and White propose castration to control prostate cancer
1903	Radium first used in treatment of cancer
1911	Peyton Rous discovers a virus that produces a sarcoma in chickens
1912	Cancer cells first grown in culture
1915	Discovery that application of coal tar to rabbits produces cancer – chemical carcinogenesis
1941	First use of a synthetic hormone to treat prostate cancer by Charles Huggins
1956	Sir Richard Doll and Austin Hill report association between tobacco and lung cancer
1964	First viral link to human cancer noted with Epstein–Barr virus
1970	David Baltimore and Howard Temin discover reverse transcriptase
1975	Cesar Milstein and George Kohler use hybridomas to produce monoclonal antibodies
1977	Development of gene sequencing techniques
1982	Oncogenes identified
1983	Tumour suppressor gene identified
1986	Lymphokine activated killer (LAK) cells used to treat advanced cancer
1989	Gene therapy used in cancer. Tumour infiltrating lymphocytes (TILs) taken from tumours, cultured and expanded with interleukin-2 and then reinjected into the patient

REFERENCES

1. Recamier JCA. Recherches sur le traitement du cancer, par les compressions methodique simple ou combinee, et sur l'histoire generale de la mime maladie. Paris: Gabon, 1829
2. Dormandy TL. In praise of peroxidation. Lancet 1988; 2:1126–1128
3. Jones ECA, Morris A. Cell biology and genetics. London: Mosby, 1999
4. Knudson AG. Stem cell regulation, tissue ontogeny, and oncogenic events. Sem Cancer Biol 1992; 3:99–106
5. Parkin JM, Morrow WJW, Pinching AJ. In: Kumar P, Clarke M (eds), Clinical medicine, 4th edn. London: WB Saunders, 1999
6. Parkinson EK. Do telomerase antagonists represent anti-cancer strategy? Br J Cancer 1996; 73:1–4
7. Raff M. Apoptosis: cell suicide for beginners. Nature 1998; 396:119
8. Wyllie AH. Apoptosis. Br Med Biol 1997; 53:451
9. Evan G, Littlewood T. Apoptosis. A matter of life and cell death. Science 1998; 281:1317–1322
10. Pignatelli M, Vessey CJ. Adhesion molecules: novel molecular tools in tumour pathology. Hum Pathol 1994; 25:849–856
11. Pignatelli M. Integrins, cadherins and catenins: molecular cross-talk in cancer cells. J Pathol 1998; 186:1–2
12. Bartek J, Lucas J, Bartkova J. Perspective: defects in cell cycle control and cancer. J Pathol 1999; 187:95–99

13. Curran S, Murray GI. Matrix metalloproteinases in tumour invasion and metastasis. J Pathol 1999; 189:300–308

14. Curran S, Murray GI. Matrix metalloproteinases: molecular aspects of their roles in tumour invasion and metastasis. Eur J Cancer 2000; 36: 1621–1630

15. Carmeliet P, Jain RK. Angiogenesis in cancer and other diseases. Nature 2000; 407:249–257

16. MacKay JA, Murray GI, MacLeod HL. Uro-oncology: a clinician's guide to immunohistochemistry. Uro-Oncology 2000; 1:11–17

17. Orkin SH. Stem cell alchemy. Nature Medicine 2000; 6:1212–1213

18. Anon. Universal amplification of DNA isolated from small regions of paraffin-embedded, formalin-fixed tissue. Biotechniques 1998; 24:47–50

19. Cheung VG, Nelson SF. Whole genome amplifications using a degenerate oligonucleotide primer allows hundreds of genotypes to be performed on less than one nanogram of genomic DNA. Proc Natl Acad Sci USA 1996; 93: 14676–14679

20. Thucydides. The history of the Peleponnesian war 2, 47–54

21. Vieweg J. The evolving role of dendritic cell therapy in urologic oncology. Curr Opin Urol 2000; 10:317

FURTHER READING

Specific aspects

Cohen HJ. Biology of aging as related to cancer. Cancer 1994; 74:2092–2110

Hahn WC, Stewart SA, Brooks MW, et al. Inhibition of telomerase limits the growth of human cancer cells. Nature Med 1999; 5:1164–1170

Hickman JA, Potten CS, Merritt AJ, Fisher TC. Apoptosis and cancer chemotherapy. Phil Trans R Soc Lond B 1994; 345:319–325

Jones PA, Ross RK. Prevention of bladder cancer. N Engl J Med 1999; 340:1424–1426

Karp JE, Chiarodo A, Brawley O, Kelloff GJ. Prostate cancer prevention: investigational approaches and opportunities. Cancer Res 1996; 56:5547–5556

London NJ, Farmery SM, Will EJ, Davison AM, Lodge JPA. Risk of neoplasia in renal transplant patients. Lancet 1995; 346:403–406

Proctor R. Cancer wars. Basic wars. New York: Basic Books, 1995

Sontag S. Illness as metaphor. New York: Penguin Books, 1983

Steele R, Lees REM, Kraus AS, Rao C. Sexual factors in the epidemiology of cancer of the prostate. J Chron Dis 1971; 24:29–37

General

Alberts B, Bray D, Lewis J, Raff M, Roberts K, Watson JD. Molecular biology of the cell, 3rd edn. London: Garland Publishing, 1994

Cotran RS, Kumar V, Collins T. Robbins pathologic basis of disease. Philadelphia: WB Saunders, 1999

Doll R, Peto R. The causes of cancer. Oxford: Oxford University Press, 1981

Duchesen GM. Principles of radiotherapy in the scientific basis of urology. In: The scientific basis of urology, Mundy AR, Fitzpatrick JM, Neill DE, George NJR (eds). Oxford: ISIS Medical Media, 1999

Franks LM, Teich NM. Introduction to the cellular and molecular biology of cancer, 3rd edn. Oxford: Oxford University Press, 1997

Lewin B. Genes VII. Oxford: Oxford University Press, 1999

Lodish H, Baltimore D, Berk A, Zipursky SL, Matsudaira P, Darnell J. Molecular cell biology, 3rd edn. Washington: Scientific Books, 1995

Mundy AR, Fitzpatrick JM, Neill DE, George NJR (eds). The scientific basis of urology. Oxford: Medical Media, 1999

Steele FGG. Basic clinical radiobiology. London: Edward Arnold, 1993

Turner PC, McLennan AG, Bates AD, White MRH. Instant notes in molecular biology. Oxford: Oxford Bios Scientific Publishers, 1997

The nervous system and cancer

Greer S. Cancer and the mind. Br J Psychiatry 1983; 143:535–543

Kowal SJ. Emotions as a cause of cancer. Psychoanal Rev 1955; 42:217–227

3

Prostate cancer

*During the last six months [IB] had suffered ...
excruciating pain in the region of the kidneys and
bladder, attended with almost constant desire to
void urine, which was effected with the greatest of
difficulty. ... An examination per rectum proved
that there existed an enlarged ... prostate gland,
and slight pressure occasioned great pain. ... The
bladder was found [at autopsy] to contain a
tumour as big as a large orange ... discovered to
derive its origin from the prostate gland. ... The
fungus plugged up both ureters ... in the liver
there were several tumours [and] several in the
lungs.*

George Langstaff[1]

*In prostatic carcinoma with marked elevation of
acid phosphatase, castration or injection of large
amounts of estrogen caused a sharp reduction of
this enzyme to or towards the normal range. ...
In 3 patients with prostatic cancer, androgen
injections caused a sharp rise of serum acid phosphatase.*

Charles Brenton Huggins, Clarence Vernard
Hodges[2]

GENERAL COMMENTARY

As men live longer, their risk of developing
prostate cancer increases. Prostate cancer is the
second greatest cancer killer of men in the
United Kingdom and is expected to become the
greatest cancer killer of men in the United
States. Until recently, men tended to present
with advanced disease, and treatment was
essentially palliative. Due to the increase in

public awareness, many countries now operate
screening systems and patients are being diagnosed at an earlier stage of disease. There is still
controversy as to whether this increases their
survival, and the absence of any large randomised control trials means that we cannot
give definitive guidance to our patients.

Intuitively, one feels that earlier treatment
should improve survival, but we have yet to
prove this.

The introduction of prostate-specific antigen
(PSA) testing has meant that patients are being
seen at a much earlier stage than previously.
This has forced us in the UK to address the
problem of early prostate cancer.

INCIDENCE

One in six American men will be affected by
clinical prostate cancer. It is the most frequently
diagnosed cancer in North American men.[3]

In the United Kingdom, prostate cancer is the
fourth most common cancer in men after cancers of the skin, lungs and large bowel, and just
over 9400 men will die from it each year.[4-6]

The incidence of new cases has risen steeply
during the last 15 years and although this may
represent a partial increase due to increasing
incidence, it will be contributed in part by better registration and an increased use of PSA
testing, which will allow earlier detection of
tumours. Once found, almost all cases will ultimately require treatment. The recent increase in
the number of consultant urologists in the UK
has also led to an increased number of

transurethral resection of prostates (TURPs) being performed which, in turn, produces case finding. More men are reaching greater ages and therefore the number of prostate cancers requiring care will inevitably rise in the next 15 years. It is estimated that, even if incidence remains steady, there will be 18,000 new cases per annum by the year 2011 in the UK.

About 16% or 1 in 6 of all men will develop clinically evident prostate cancer in life. At postmortem, a pathological diagnosis of the disease can be made in up to 30% of men over the age of 50. Many cancers of prostate may be latent or clinically irrelevant, but follow-up of many such patients indicates that, for many, it proves to be a fatal condition.[6]

The lowest incidence rates of cancer of the prostate (CAP) have been observed in Asian, Japanese and Chinese populations. Migration studies suggest that men tend to take on the risk of their host country. There is no published evidence of increased risk in Asian, Chinese or Afro-Caribbean UK communities.[7,8]

The incidence of cancer of the prostate is shown in Table 3.1 and incidence, mortality and survival in Figure 3.1.

DIFFERENT BEHAVIOUR OF PROSTATE CANCERS

Prostate cancer may exist in two forms: a latent form and a clinically evident form characterised by relentless progress if unchecked. It is not understood what influences potential changes from an apparently latent to an aggressive disease and the process is probably a multistep one.[10,11]

MORTALITY

The relative survival rates for several countries are listed in Table 3.2.

AETIOLOGY – NON-GENETIC

A wide variety of causes for prostate cancer have been suggested. There have been many debates about increased sexual activity being a factor, the hypothesis being that a viral or similar agent has triggered these cancers. No evidence of any strength has been obtained to support these theories, however.

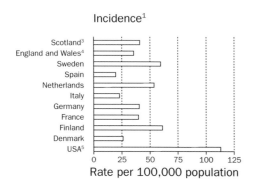
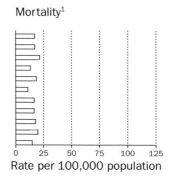
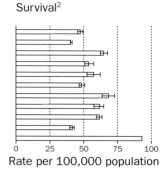

1 Age-standardised rates per 100,000 person-years at risk (World standard population) 1995.
2 Relative survival at 5 years, patients diagnosed 1985–89.

3 Scotland: survival, ages 15–99.
4 England and Wales: incidence 1993; mortality 1995; survival 1986–90 (ages 15–99).
5 USA (SEER, whites): incidence and mortality 1992–96; survival 1989–95.

Figure 3.1 International comparison of incidence, mortality and survival (with 95% CI all ages).

Table 3.1 Age-standardized incidence rates and standard errors per 100,000 for cancer of prostate (ICD-9 185)[9]

Country	Incidence	Standard error
US, SEER:[a] Black	137.0	1.64
US, Hawaii: White	108.2	3.48
US, SEER: White	100.8	0.40
Canada	64.7	0.27
US, Hawaii: Japanese	64.2	2.09
US, Hawaii: Chinese	62.9	4.44
Zimbabwe, Harare: European	55.7	7.03
Sweden	55.3	0.37
US, Puerto Rico	54.7	0.82
South Australia	53.6	1.02
Austria, Tyrol	51.6	1.66
France, Calvados	50.5	1.59
US, Hawaii: Filipino	49.5	2.83
US, Hawaii: Hawaiian	42.1	2.09
Finland	41.3	0.46
The Netherlands	39.6	0.31
Germany: Saarland	35.9	0.96
Brazil, Goiania	35.2	2.08
Uruguay, Montevideo	32.6	1.09
UK, Scotland	31.2	0.40
Denmark	31.0	0.38
Ireland, Southern	30.9	1.28
Zimbabwe, Harare: African	29.2	3.07
UK, England and Wales	28.0	0.15
Italy, Genoa	24.7	0.83
Czech Republic	24.1	0.27
Israel: All Jews	23.9	0.45
Germany: Eastern States	23.7	0.36
Ecuador, Quito	22.4	2.08
Spain, Zaragoza	19.7	0.75
Peru, Lima	19.4	0.71
Kuwait: non-Kuwaitis	18.3	3.64
Philippines, Manila	17.6	0.71
Argentina, Concordia	16.2	2.40
Poland, Warsaw City	15.7	0.6
Yugoslavia, Vojvodina	14.7	0.47
Japan, Hiroshima	10.9	0.62
Israel: non-Jews	10.4	1.12
Singapore: Chinese	9.8	0.49
Hong Kong	7.9	0.24
India, Bombay	7.9	0.30
Kuwait: Kuwaitis	6.5	1.13
China, Shanghai	2.3	0.10
Vietnam: Hanoi	1.2	0.2
Korea, Kangwa	0.9	0.52

[a]SEER = Surveillance, Epidemiology and End Results programme.

Table 3.2 International comparison of survival from prostate cancer (ICD-9 185).[9] Relative survival (%) at 5 years, all ages, patients diagnosed 1985–89

Country	Survival rate (%)
USA	93.1
Germany	69.0
Sweden	65.0
Finland	62.0
France	62.0
Netherlands	58.0
Spain	54.0
Italy	49.0
Scotland	48.1
Denmark	42.0
England and Wales	41.0

The only areas of particular interest are those of exposure to metals, such as cadmium, and the association of prostate cancer with countries with a high meat intake: the hypothesis being that animal fats predispose to cancer.[12–14]

However, animal fats may be a proxy indicator for our Western lifestyle. Of course, survival is greater in Western countries in any case, and by the time that these factors have been corrected, the associations are not so impressive.

CARCINOGENESIS

Carcinogenesis in prostate cancer is believed to be a multistep process involving initiation, promotion and progression:[10]

- primary prevention procedures are intended to prevent initiation
- secondary prevention attempts to remove or affect promoting factors
- tertiary prevention is designed to affect preneoplastic lesions, such as prostatic intraepithelial neoplasia (PIN).[3]

Many foods of plant origin contain isoflavonoids, flavonoids and ligans. They possess weak oestrogenic activity but become transformed by intestinal bacteria to produce phytoestrogens, which have stronger oestrogenic activity.

Selenium

There is at present a trial in Arizona involving 974 men with a history of skin cancer. They have been given a daily supplement of 200 μg selenium or placebo for a mean of 4.5 years and follow up for 6.5 years, with no difference in the incidence of skin cancer, but there has been an observed 63% reduction in prostate cancer.[3]

CHEMOPREVENTION OF CAP

5α-reductase inhibitors

Testosterone is converted to dihydrotestosterone in the prostate by 5α-reductase. Finasteride is a 5α-reductase inhibitor. There is at present an American control trial of 18,000 healthy men, over the age of 55, who are randomised to receive either 5 mg of oral finasteride daily or placebo. At 7 years, all survivors will undergo sextant biopsies. This trial will not achieve maturity until 2004.[12]

In Finland a chemoprevention trial, using α-tocopherol or vitamin E, plus β-carotene was conducted in 29,000 heavy smokers, treated for periods between 5 and 8 years. Lung cancer incidence was not reduced, but rather increased by 18% in the treated group, but a 30% reduction of prostate cancer was noted.[3]

Inherited deficiency of 5α-reductase

Men with an uncommon inherited deficiency of 5α-reductase have normal testosterone levels and develop secondary sexual characteristics at puberty. Their prostates are underdeveloped, and benign prostatic hyperplasia (BPH) and prostate cancer are not seen in this group of men.[8]

RISK FACTORS FOR PROSTATE CANCER

Obesity

Obese men appear to have a relative risk of 1.25 (to 1). Gronberg and his colleagues found that total food consumption is related to an increase in prostate cancer risk and that body mass index (BMI) was related. Diet may affect hormone levels, and this was seen in the urinary steroid levels in black South African men given a Western diet.[15,16]

Vitamin A intake

Men with an extremely high intake of vitamin A suffer an increased risk of developing prostate cancer.[17]

Sexual activity

The evidence that hormonal levels in men with prostate cancer are different is a tempting hypothesis, but unproven, because of the long time between measurement of hormonal levels in early youth and the development of prostate cancer; therefore, data can be very misleading.[18]

Nuclear power

Rooney and his colleagues investigated 136 nuclear plant employees and found that they had a 2.36 times higher risk of developing prostate cancer, with respect to a control population. It was felt that the risk factors were supposedly exposure to tritiated chromium, iron, cobalt and possibly zinc.[19]

Androgen and steroid receptors

Genetic polymorphism is an expression of steroid receptors and may modify risk in prostate cancer, particularly after androgen stimulation.

Long CAG repeats in exon-1 of the androgen receptor gene on the X-chromosome may have a protective role against androgen overstimulation.[20]

Luteinizing hormone releasing hormone (LH RH) agonists and insulin-like growth factor

It has been observed that LH RH agonists interfere with the mitogenic activity of the insulin-like growth factor system in androgen-independent prostate cancer cells.[21]

Deprivation

Carstairs and his colleague produced an index of deprivation in Scotland and showed a positive correlation between deprivation and prostate cancer incidence, but this work has yet to be verified.[22]

AETIOLOGY – GENETIC FACTORS FOR PROSTATE CANCER

It has been estimated that 9% of all cases of CAP can be attributed to genetic causes, and that this figure increases to 45% in men diagnosed in the under-55 group. As work on the human genome proceeds, more and more genes are being discovered with the relationship to disease: 43% of early onset prostate cancer in men under 55 years of age occurs in certain gene carriers.[21,22] In families with three or more first-degree relatives, an affected locus has been identified on chromosome 1q24–25.

There would appear to be an association with the *BRCA*-1 (breast cancer) gene. It is known that males who carry a mutation in the *BRCA*-1 gene have an increased risk of prostate cancer, and it may be that there is some benefit of offering such males screening.

The difficulty of examining these as aetiological agents is due to the nature of cancer itself. As cancer becomes less differentiated, a degree of chaos creeps into the genome and, in general, the further cancer is along its course, the more disorganised its nucleus and its DNA become.[23–26]

Risk

Risk increases with the following factors.

The number of affected relatives
- 1 affected gives a 2-fold increase
- 2 affected gives a 5-fold increase
- 3 affected gives an 11-fold increased risk.

Age at presentation
A 17-fold increase in risk is seen where a brother is affected between 45 and 50 years of age (Table 3.3).[24]

CLINICAL PRESENTATION

Early prostate cancer does not itself have symptoms, and only when the prostate cancer expands does it give notice of its presence. Most tumours arise in the peripheral zone, which is remote from the urethra. Although local extension into the ejaculatory duct may lead to a loss in ejaculatory volume and haemospermia, these symptoms are very rare as presenting features.

Digital rectal examination (DRE)

This examination is often neglected or performed poorly. It demands experience of the examiner and an appreciation of what and what cannot be discerned.

Size
The size of a prostate can be estimated rectally using a well-lubricated gloved forefinger in the patient's rectum. One pitfall is to overestimate prostatic size, being deceived by a full bladder or one which is not emptying. An experienced urologist uses DRE as one estimate of prostatic size to determine therapy, and to decide on TURP versus an open prostatectomy.

Consistency
Consistency is the key to determining clinical presence of carcinoma. Although most carcinomas occur posteriorly, it is possible to miss at least 50% of carcinomas, especially early ones. It is possible to feel nodules which require biopsy. With experience, it is possible to distinguish between nodular BPH and potentially malignant lesions.

A normal prostate has a smooth consistency, with a well-preserved median sulcus. Carcinomas are hard, almost like bone, and are usually non-tender. Tenderness may indicate prostatitis, but this can coexist with cancer.

Coley and his colleagues reviewed 25 publications on the effectiveness of primary DRE.[27] There were no controlled studies and no evidence that one-time or repeated DRE reduced the rates of morbidity or mortality attributed to prostate cancer. They concluded that it had a positive predictive value of 15%, but had an overall cancer detection rate of 2%.

These studies were performed in a primary care setting. Many family physicians/GPs are

---

Table 3.3 Estimated risk ratios for prostate cancer in first-degree relatives of cases, by age at onset in case and additional affected family members. The hazard ratio is shown, with 95% CI in brackets[24]

Age at onset of case	No additional relatives affected	One or more additional first-degree relatives affected
50	1.9 (1.2–2.8)	7.1 (3.7–13.6)
60	1.4 (1.1–1.7)	5.2 (3.1–8.7)
70	1.0	3.8 (2.4–6.0)

Table 3.4 Estimated likelihood ratios for results on digital rectal examination (DRE). Abnormality was defined as asymmetry, induration or nodularity

Result on digital rectal examination and study (Reference)	Likelihood ratio	
	Intracapsular tumour	Extracapsular tumour
Suspicious		
Chodak et al.[30]	1.5	8.6
Richie et al.[29]	2.0	2.7
Non-suspicious		
Chodak et al.[28]	0.96	0.53
Richie et al.[29]	0.83	0.72

unfamiliar with rectal examination and, although it is possible to detect an advanced T3/T4 cancer, this is hardly contributory if we are attempting to pick up early disease which is amenable to radical treatment. DRE tends to detect peripheral zone cancer. In patients with PSA-detected tumour, around half of the detected cases were found adjacent to the peripheral zone capsule.[28]

Coley found two volunteer studies (Table 3.4) which provided age-stratified data to determine the operating characteristics for DRE in the detection of pathologically confined and unconfined prostate cancer. This is found to have a positive predictive value of 15% in the first study by Scardino and Catalona.[29] There was found to be positive predictive value in 26% in the second study by Chodak et al.[30]

Coley then went on to estimate that a suspicious DRE increases the odds of an intracapsular tumour larger than 0.5 ml to twofold, and the odds of an extracapsular tumour are increased from 2.7 to 8.6-fold.

Prostate-specific antigen

Patients are often discovered by an increase in PSA (Table 3.5) and, at a slightly later stage, may be discovered with both an increase in PSA and a palpable nodule at DRE.

PSA is a serine protease, i.e. an enzyme that breaks down a protein at a point where the protein has the amino acid serine in its sequence – serine proteases are a family of which other members are chymotrypsin, trypsin and thrombin. PSA is composed of glycoprotein: a combination of a sugar and a protein. PSA has a role in semen liquefaction, which is known to be important in animals, but its precise role in humans is obscure. Purification was generally attributed to Wang and his colleagues.[31] Despite being first identified in 1970, it was not until 1987 that Stamey produced his groundbreaking paper, documenting the relationship between PSA and clinical prognosis, that the clinical significance of PSA was made.[32] The half-life of PSA in serum is between 2 and 3 days; thus, PSA levels should not be estimated for at least 2

Table 3.5 Chances of prostate cancer at various prostate-specific antigen (PSA) levels[35]

PSA level	Chance of prostate cancer
<4 ng/ml	1:50
4.0–10.0 ng/ml	1:4
>10.0 ng/ml	between 1:2 and 2:3

weeks after radical prostatectomy. Finasteride, a specific inhibitor of the enzyme 5α-reductase, which converts testosterone to dihydrotestosterone, lowers PSA by 50% after 1 year of treatment. PSA is found in increasing levels with age in sera of men. It is found free and also bound to antiproteases such as α_1-antichymotrypsin.[33,34]

International variations in the incidence of CAP in recent years are highly influenced by differences in the use and availability of the PSA test. It is believed that more than 50% of men in the USA aged over 50 years have had their PSA tested.[36]

There have been various attempts to increase the predictive value of PSA testing.

1. Age adjustment
Reference levels are banded, e.g.

40–50 years	0–2.5 ng/ml
51–60	0–3.5 ng/ml
61–70	0–4.5 ng/ml
70+	0–6.5 ng/ml

The upper limit of normal is increased with age.[35]

2. PSA density
PSA levels can be adjusted against the measured prostatic volume on ultrasound. In men with a PSA level of >4 ng/ml, a density of greater than 0.15 has a higher risk of cancer.

3. PSA velocity
Incremental changes of greater than 0.75 ng/ml over a 2-year period are associated with an increased risk of cancer.

4. Free to total PSA
Men with prostate cancer have a greater proportion of bound PSA to free PSA. The risk varies at different PSA levels:

Total PSA <4.0 ng/ml	0.19
Total PSA 4–10 ng/ml	0.24

Ratio levels which fall at, or below, the above cut-off levels suggest further investigation may be indicated.

Other forms of PSA such as membrane-associated PSA are being investigated but are not in wide use at present.[37,38] Factors affecting PSA level are listed in Table 3.6.

Patients with elevated levels are investigated by transrectal ultrasound and biopsy if appropriate. Diagnosis by this means leads to the allocation of a specific stage – T1c (tumour identified by needle biopsy).

Four studies where volunteers have been used have been identified. This provided age distributions and allowed Coley and his colleagues to compute likelihood ratios for several ranges of PSA levels (Table 3.7).

Repeated testing increases the likelihood that detected tumours will be pathologically organ confined and therefore amenable to radical treatment.[44]

Transrectal ultrasound and biopsy (TRUS)

Transrectal ultrasound uses high-frequency sound waves from a transducer which transmits and receives these sound waves and is able to convert the pattern of reflectance into a picture. The clarity of the picture is referred to as its resolution.

Table 3.6 Factors affecting prostate-specific antigen (PSA) level

Result	Condition or activity causing change in PSA
Rise	Prostate cancer
Rise	Benign prostatic hyperplasia
Rise	Prostate biopsy
Rise	Prostatitis (usually caused by infection)
Rise	Prostate manipulation (i.e. DRE or TRUS)
Rise	Cycling! (controversial)
Decrease	Hormone therapy
Decrease	Prostatectomy (removal of prostate)
Variable	Sex
Variable	Exercise

DRE = digital rectal examination;
TRUS = transurethral ultrasound.

Table 3.7   Estimated likelihood ratios for results of PSA testing[39–42]

Study (reference and PSA level)	Likelihood ratio	
	Intracapsular tumour	Extracapsular ratio
Catalona et al[39] and Brawer et al:[40]		
<4.0 ng/ml	0.98	0.09
4.1–10 ng/ml	1.4	5.1
>10 ng/ml	0.4	49.6
Richie et al:[41]		
<4.0 ng/ml	0.7	0.4
>4.1 ng/ml	3.0	4.6
Catalona et al:[42]		
<4.0 ng/ml	0.8	0.5
4.1–10 ng/ml	2.8	3.2
>10 ng/ml	3.0	23.7

TRUS is able to detect twice as many cancers as DRE in a screened population, but the sensitivity and specificity are low. Colour Doppler is not believed at present to improve detection rates.

The main value of TRUS is to identify suspicious areas and then to guide biopsies of these suspicious areas.

Most small cancers have a hypoechoic appearance, but larger tumours may have a mixed hypo- and hyperechoic pattern. About one-third of tumours have an isoechoic pattern, and biopsies may be picking up tumour by random sampling of prostate tissue.

Biopsy

Ultrasound-assisted biopsy using 18G biopsies of the prostate are used routinely and the use of a spring-assisted needle is recommended.

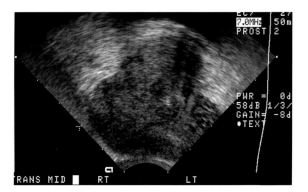

Figure 3.2 Prostate cancer mass protruding anteriorly (TOP) from peripheral zone: biopsy positive.

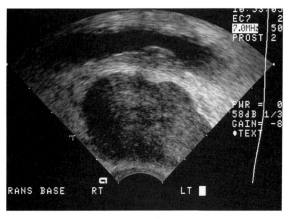

Figure 3.3 Prostate cancer. Same patient, inferior view.

It is less painful for the patient and allows a quick and accurate biopsy. Antibiotic cover is mandatory, and particular care should be taken with patients with prostheses such as artificial hips or heart valves, ensuring that antibiotic levels are high at the time of biopsy, by using intravenous broad-spectrum agents or by giving them at least 1 hour prior to biopsy.[45,46]

Biopsies are principally aimed at suspicious areas, but if there is no localising feature, sextant biopsies are obtained.[47]

It is becoming more common to direct these sextant biopsies laterally to increase the yield of cancer and to allow more effective information about curative potential of major surgery.[48]

Now, even more than six biopsies are commonly performed, and local anaesthetic may be infiltrated into the neurovascular bundle.

CLASSIFICATION OF PROSTATE CANCER STAGE

The TNM (tumour, node, metastases) staging system for prostate cancers is shown in Table 3.8. It is compared with the Whitmore–Jewett system in Tables 3.9 and 3.10.

The European Association of Urology (EAU) guidelines on staging are of interest.

T stage

T staging of prostate cancer is based on DRE and imaging studies.

N stage

Lymph node status (N stage) is only of importance where curative treatment is anticipated. Accurate lymph node status (N stage) can only be determined by bilateral pelvic lymphadenectomy and histological analysis. Computed tomography/magnetic resonance imaging (CT/MR) are of limited value due to low sensitivity but may be used to guide aspiration biopsies.

Table 3.8   TNM staging of prostate cancer[49,50]

Stage	Finding
T1	Not palpable or visible
T1a	<5% of tissue resected at TURP infiltrated by cancer
T1b	>5% of tissue resected at TURP infiltrated by cancer
T1c	Needle biopsy
T2	Confined within prostate
T2a	One lobe
T2b	Both lobes
T3	Through prostatic capsule
T3a	Extracapsular
T3b	Seminal vesicle(s)
T4	Fixed or invades adjacent structures: bladder neck, external sphincter, rectum, levator muscles, pelvic wall
N1	Regional lymph node(s)
M1a	Non-regional lymph node(s)
M1b	Bone(s)
M1c	Other site(s)

TURP = transurethal resection of prostate.

Table 3.9   TNM versus Whitmore–Jewett classifications for prostate cancer stage

TNM	Whitmore–Jewett
T1	A
T1, T2	A1
T2, T3	A2
T2	B
T2a, T2b	B1
T2c	B2
T3	C
T3a, T3b	C1
T3c	C2
M1 + N1	D

TNM	Whitmore-Jewett	TNM definition
		Tumour found incidentally, usually during transurethral resection of the prostate, and:
T1a	A1	<5% of tissue is prostate cancer
T1b	A2	>5% of tissue is prostate cancer
T1c	B0	Tumour identified during prostate-specific antigen test, with no other clinical signs
		Tumour detectable by digital rectal examination, but confined within the prostate and with involvement of:
T2a	B1	no more than one-half of a single lobe
T2b	B2	more than one-half of a single lobe
T2c	B3	both lobes
		Tumour extends through and beyond the prostate capsule, with:
T3a	C1	unilateral extracapsular extension
T3b	C1	bilateral extracapsular extension
T3c	C2–3	invasion of one or both of the seminal vesicles
		Tumour localised to the pelvic region, but:
T4a		invades bladder neck and/or external sphincter and/or rectum
T4b		invades levator muscles and/or is fixed to pelvic wall
N+	D1	Prostate cancer evident in pelvic lymph nodes or extends into the rectal area
	D1.5	Rising prostate-specific antigen level after failed local therapy
M+	D2	Prostate cancer evident outside the pelvic area, usually as metastases
	D2.5	Rising prostate-specific antigen after a nadir induced by adequate hormonal therapy
	D3	(Tumour no longer responsive to hormonal therapy)

Table 3.10 Stages of prostate cancer: a comparison of the TNM and Whitmore–Jewett systems

There is no D3 equivalent in the TNM system and no T4 equivalent in the Whitmore–Jewett system.[49,50]

M stage

Skeletal metastases are best assessed by a bone scan. This may not be indicated in asymptomatic patients if the serum PSA level is less than 10 ng/ml in the presence of well or moderately differentiated tumours.[51,52] The Whitmore-Jewett classification is used more in the USA and can be seen in Tables 3.9 and 3.10.

SCREENING FOR PROSTATE CANCER

Despite many surgeons pressing for screening, there is reluctance to introduce it in many countries. In the United States, men are assessed similarly, although there is no systematic screening. Certain states have introduced a limited form of screening, but at present most of the screening, which is operating worldwide, is an extension of case finding.

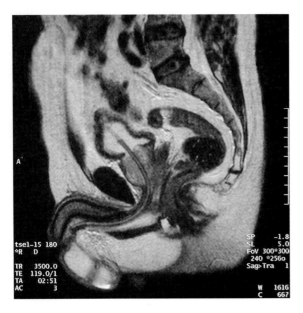

Figure 3.4 Sagittal T2 MR image of mid-line CAP. Note catheter in situ and prostate tumour with extracapsular invasion.

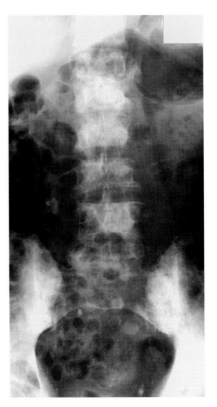

Figure 3.5 Typical sclerotic metastases (L1, L2 and L4) from primary prostatic cancer.

The difficulties of introducing mass screening are partly due to cost, and many governments really do not wish to address the question of early prostate cancer.

The dearth of clinical trials in early prostate cancer – to show that there is clear survival benefit – has hampered the case for the introduction of screening. In the USA, where, historically, treatment has been more aggressive than in the UK, the death rate from prostate cancer has gone down despite an increasing incidence. Surgeons attribute this to early surgery. Screening can be defined as the performance of an observation or a test(s) in apparently well patients to detect unrecognised disease at a stage at which an intervention can significantly modify the natural history and outcome of the disease.

The aim of screening is to reduce morbidity and mortality from disease, by its detection and treatment before symptoms appear.

Ten general principles of screening, first set down in 1968, are:

1. The condition should pose an important health problem.
2. The natural history of the disease should be well understood.
3. There should be a recognisable early stage.
4. Treatment of the disease in early stage should be of more benefit than treatment started at a later stage.
5. There should be a suitable test.
6. The test should be acceptable to the population.
7. There should be adequate facilities for the diagnosis and treatment of the abnormalities detected.
8. For diseases of insidious onset, screening should be repeated at intervals, determined by the natural history of the disease.
9. The chance of physical or psychological

harm to those screened should be less than the chance of benefit.

10. The cost of the screening programme should be balanced against the benefit it provides.

When one examines the criteria of screening against prostate cancer, many of the criteria are more than fulfilled.

Screening for prostate cancer involves the examination of asymptomatic men, firstly by DRE and a blood test for PSA.[53-55]

There is debate as to the desirability of including DRE at the initial screen. Although its use will increase the number of cancers detected, there is some evidence that DRE may miss life-threatening tumours. Although in two general practice studies in the UK, DRE and PSA were acceptable to members of the general male population, it has been found in larger pilot studies in Belgium and the Netherlands that acceptance rates may be as low as 35–40% when both tests were used. Acceptance rates in UK males of screening for other diseases by blood tests are of a higher order, up to 60%. In PSA-based screening programmes, over 97% of cancers detected on initial evaluation are clinically localised to the prostate. The case for screening would therefore appear to be strong; but the most important objection, however, is that there have been no randomised control trials with sufficient power to detect any improvement in mortality from medical intervention. Finally, and probably most importantly, there is lack of true evidence-based information regarding the effect of treatment from early prostate cancer.

Those men with a suspicious DRE or a raised PSA are then investigated by an ultrasound carried out transrectally (TRUS) and biopsy where indicated, either systematically on quadrants of the prostate and/or of suspicious areas. The disease is then confirmed histologically. Men that have the disease can then be staged and offered treatment, such as radical prostatectomy or radical radiotherapy, or be monitored by watchful waiting until they develop symptoms.

Screening for prostate cancer has operated in Germany since 1978, and rectal examination is included in insurance annual check ups in Belgium. In France, worksite PSA screening has been launched by occupational health services for men aged between 50 and 65 years of age. The United States National Cancer Institute has stated that there is insufficient evidence to establish that a decrease in mortality from prostate cancer occurs, with screening by DRE, TRUS or serum marker, and yet the American Urological Association and the American Cancer Society have published guidelines advocating annual DRE and PSA testing for men over the age of 50.

Bias

There have been a number of small screening studies, but they have relied on volunteers willing to respond to invitations to screening, and this immediately introduced selection bias. Two other forms of bias which can occur in screening studies are those of lead-time bias and length-time bias.

Lead-time bias occurs when asymptomatic tumours are detected earlier by screening programmes and this earlier detection does not affect the course of the disease. The cancers that are confined to the prostate can be slow growing and may be biologically insignificant as far as the patient is concerned. This naturally makes the screen population appear to survive longer and have a higher proportion of early disease, independent of any surgical or medical intervention.

Length-time bias occurs because asymptomatic tumours detected may grow slower than tumours which are symptomatic, once again having the above effects. These effects occur in the absence of any real improvement in mortality.[56,57]

Characteristics of tumours detected

Seventy per cent of tumours detected through screening are organ-confined and could potentially be eradicated by radical prostatectomy. This eradication is defined as undetectable PSA levels for up to 10 years after surgery.

More slowly growing or latent tumours may be more likely to be detected by screening, but might have a longer preclinical course. The rate of detection of these tumours would increase if the screen is applied over a number of years. Fenely reviewed the characteristics of tumours found at screening and concluded that clinically important disease is indeed identified by a screening process.[58]

General morbidity associated with screening

Another factor which must be addressed before the introduction of screening is that of the morbidity of screening. Unnecessary anxiety may be induced by screening, especially for the high proportion of men found to have a falsely positive initial result.

A combination of PSA and DRE screening results in the detection rate of 4–6%, but this means that 20% of the screened population will require biopsy. Putting it another way, 4 or 5 men must undergo biopsy to find a single case of prostate cancer. If PSA is used without DRE, only 3 patients must undergo biopsy to find one case of prostate cancer.

Specific risks of screening

The test DRE is unlikely to produce any significant detriment to the patient and nor is the venepuncture used to perform the PSA test. A TRUS on its own is hardly more significant than a DRE; however, there is a 2% infection rate with a TRUS biopsy.[45,46]

Further evaluation of a false-positive test would in turn expose the patient to further anxiety, and the risks of the biopsy.

Anxiety
The whole question of anxiety induced by the diagnosis of cancer, and occasionally of being given a clean bill of health, is difficult to evaluate. The issue of informed consent requires to be addressed. There is a risk that a patient found to have an early cancer would find it difficult to either gain life assurance or would be given punitive rates. The risk of avoiding health cover is nonexistent in the UK, unless one includes the difficulty in obtaining private health cover.

Prostate cancer support groups are beginning to question whether men and their diseases receive as much attention as they deserve, particularly when compared with breast or cervical cancer, and such sexist arguments are beginning to be voiced. There is not sufficient evidence to introduce screening widely, but clinical trials of screening are required to assess the efficacy of screening.

The absence of data to support prostatic screening does not mean such a benefit may not exist. There is an urgent need for evaluation of the benefits of a screening programme but this is not known. The appropriate interval between screening is unknown and the benefits conveyed by a screening programme may not balance the cost of such intervention.[59–67]

PATHOLOGY

Prostate cancer may exist in two forms: a latent form and a clinically evident form characterised by relentless progress if unchecked. It is not understood what influences potential changes from an apparently latent to an aggressive disease and the process is probably a multistep one.[10,11]

McNeal[68] has proposed a division of the prostate into zones, and this has achieved widespread acceptance.

- *Anterior:* The anterior portion has no glandular tissue and is composed of fibromuscular stroma.
- *Central:* The central portion is composed of the transition zone, lying above and on both sides of the verumontanum, and the periurethral tissue. This is the zone which enlarges in benign prostatic hyperplasia.
- *Peripheral:* This totally comprises glandular tissue, and represents two-thirds of the total gland volume in the young male.

Most tumours arise from the acinar epithelium of the peripheral zone of the prostate: 95% are adenocarcinomas, and arise from the acinar or ductal epithelium of the prostate and are usually composed of small glandular acini that infiltrate in an irregular haphazard manner. The critical feature is the absence of the basal cell layer. Keratin 34β E12 stains the basal cell layer and this stain can be used in diagnosis.[69,70]

Mucinous and ductal carcinomas have a worse prognosis than adenocarcinomas.

Eighty-five per cent of tumours are multifocal. Perineural infiltration is one of the hallmarks of diagnosis of infiltrative lesions but does not of itself carry a worse prognosis.[60] C-*erb*-2 in early tumours is associated with a worse prognosis.[25] The *Rb* (retinoblastoma) gene is absent or decreased in CAP, suggesting that its loss may be an early event in CAP.[26]

Overexpression of the p53 gene is found in increasing proportion in more advanced disease, suggesting that it is a late event.[71]

The bcl-2 protein has been found in all primary and metastatic carcinomas which have become hormonally resistant. Changes in the androgen receptor have also been noted in this group.

Androgen receptor

The androgen receptor (AR) produces an external male phenotype when exposed to androgens. Androgens are required to produce virilisation of wolffian duct structures, the urogenital sinus and the genital tubercle.[72]

Although androgen binding to the AR is the usual method of AR activation, it has been shown that AR-mediated transcription is influenced 'downstream' by cytoplasmic signalling cross-talk or nucleoprotein cross-modulation.[73]

Androgen-regulated gene activity, after androgen ablation, may hold the key to new therapy for hormone relapsed prostate cancer.[73]

Dysplasia or PIN?

The term 'intraductal dysplasia' was first used in 1986 and this led to a grading system of mild, moderate and severe dysplasia. Because of con-troversy, however, the term prostatic intraepithelial neoplasia (PIN) was proposed as a synonym for intraductal dysplasia and these roughly correspond to mild, moderate and severe dysplasia. Although there are inconsistencies, the term high grade is used only for PIN3.

PIN1 – McNeill stated: 'There is not a sharp line of demarcation between grade 1 dysplasia and mild degrees of deviation from a normal histology.' PIN1 is normally not commented on in pathological reports.[74]

PIN2 – Often PIN2 exists with PIN3.

PIN3. At low magnification, high-grade PIN has a basal filling appearance. This is caused by enlarged nuclei, hyperchromatism, over mapping nuclei and epithelial hyperplasia. The first form of PIN that is identified is nuclear atypia. In these cases the basal cell is still visible and it is difficult to distinguish between atypical and normal nuclei. In a more advanced high-grade PIN, micropapillary projections and cribriform (perforated with small apertures like a sieve) patterns emerge. Peripheral nuclei tend to be more flamboyant when located against the basement membrane. These peripherally located nuclei were used to distinguish the various groups of PIN.

High-grade PIN is assumed to be a precursor in some forms of carcinoma. Some authors believe that PIN3 should be termed carcinoma in situ or intraductal carcinoma, but the natural history of PIN is unknown. There are concerns that patients may be overtreated if PINs 1 and 2 are reported but PIN3 is a signal to the pathologist to look harder in the specimen since it commonly coexists with overt cancer.[75,76]

Studies have been started by the National Institutes of Health to use finasteride to assess whether PIN can be decreased and may thus be used as a chemopreventative agent in adenocarcinoma of the prostate.[3]

The Gleason system

The standard histological grading system is that developed by Gleason[77] who graded prostate cancer in a hierarchical way, starting with grade 1, in which the tumour is arranged in an almost recognisable glandular

Differentiation

Grade

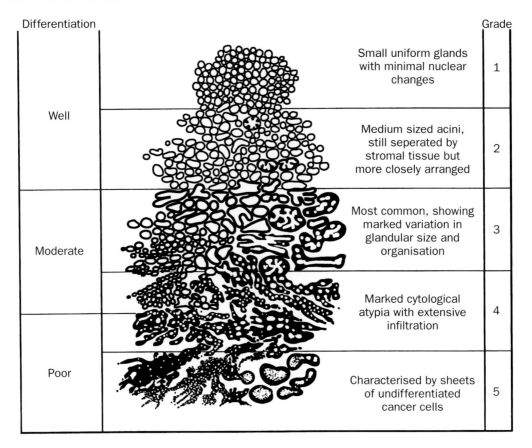

	Small uniform glands with minimal nuclear changes	1
Well	Medium sized acini, still seperated by stromal tissue but more closely arranged	2
Moderate	Most common, showing marked variation in glandular size and organisation	3
	Marked cytological atypia with extensive infiltration	4
Poor	Characterised by sheets of undifferentiated cancer cells	5

Figure 3.6 Gleason scoring system for prostate cancer.

structure (Figure 3.6). In grade 5, the tumours show sheets of undifferentiated cancer cells. Grade 2 tumours show medium-sized glands, still separated by stromal tissue. Grade 3 tumours, which are the most common, show marked variation and glandular size and organisation and generally show infiltration of the stroma and neighbouring tissues. Grade 4 tumours show marked cytological atypia, with extensive infiltration. Grade 5 tumours show an undifferentiated appearance.

Prostate cancers, when examined microscopically, consist of various different areas. To obtain a representative histology, Gleason proposed a system of scoring, adding together the sum of the two most prominent grades observed at low power. These correspond to a 10-year likelihood of local progression of 25% in a Gleason score of 4 or less (well differentiated); about 50% in Gleason scores 5–7, which are moderately differentiated; and a 75% likelihood of progression in tumours where the score is 8 or more.

Histological changes occur with hormonal treatment, and Gleason becomes unreliable after hormonal therapy: 0.5% of patients may not show cancer after hormonal treatment, the so-called vanishing cancers.

NATURAL HISTORY OF PROSTATE CANCER

In the past, age and common co-morbidity of prostate cancer patients, allied with a slow rate of growth in many tumours, resulted in relatively conservative policies of surveillance. Conservative treatment is also referred to as expectant treatment, watchful waiting, or active monitoring.

The second term is used to acknowledge that treatment will be given on an ad hoc basis when or if required. Carter and colleagues take a more robust view of these options calling them treatment with no curative intent.[86]

Despite the wealth of literature on prostate cancer (over 7000 publications between 1996 and 1999), there remains uncertainty about the clinical course of prostate cancer in all patients.

In older men with lower life expectancy, independent of their prostate cancer, conservative treatment is favoured if the disease is asymptomatic.

The debate focuses on the efficacy of treatment and the morbidity of any such treatment.

About 16% or 1 in 6 of all men will develop clinically evident prostate cancer in life, although the prevalence of undiagnosed prostate cancer is known to be high in the elderly; data are much poorer in younger men.

To assess the natural history of untreated disease, we must rely on observational studies.[78]

George[79] in the UK reported a prospective study in 1988. He followed, prospectively, 120 patients with early-localised cancer. They were elderly with a mean age of 74.8 years. All had histological confirmed disease and negative bone scans. Local tumour progressed in 100 patients, but metastases developed in only 13. Actuarial survival was 80% at 5 years and 75% at 7 years (excluding non-cancer deaths). He makes the point that earlier investigators lacked bone scans and could not distinguish metastatic disease accurately. It was also pointed out that earlier studies included patients in the non-treatment arm if they were too old or too ill.

Johansson[80–82] reported a series of 229 patients in 1989 with T0–2 tumours of all grades. They reported 37% deaths at follow up, with only 7% from CAP.

In 1992, at least 4 studies of early CAP were reported. Adolfsson et al[83] reported 122 patients followed prospectively and given deferred treatment. Most patients had low-volume tumours, but a number of patients with larger tumour who did not wish treatment were included. At 5 years, only 2 patients were dead from CAP and 21 had died from other illnesses; 99 were alive. They computed the risk of dying from CAP was 1% at 5 years and 16% at 10 years.[83]

Johansson reported further on his series, with 16 fewer patients, i.e. 223 patients with early untreated CAP: 8.5% died from CAP at a mean follow up of 123 months. Of the total of 124 deaths, 105 (85%) were reckoned to be from other causes. In a subgroup considered eligible for (but not given or wishing) radical surgery, the progression free 10-year survival rate was 53.1%.[82]

Jones[84] reviewed 233 patients with stages A or B CAP who had conservative management. He felt that the probability of survival of the total cohort was comparable with similarly aged US males. He makes the point that surveillance requires patient compliance and attendance. Since the advent of PSA, and TRUS: 'determination of progression and/or activity of the disease (occurs) significantly earlier than waiting for the patient to register pain, weight loss, or lethargy.'

Aus[85] examined retrospectively a series of 503 patients with a diagnosis of prostate cancer. In patients with no metastases at diagnosis and who survived more than 10 years, 63% died from prostate cancer. In men aged less than 65 years, at diagnosis, 75% died from prostate cancer.

Many of these reported series were prior to PSA and the staging of disease may be in doubt. In an attempt to address this, Carter et al[86] measured PSA in normal and men with BPH, localised or malignant prostates using sera stored for an average of 17 years prior to diagnosis. Men with final metastatic disease had PSA levels significantly greater than controls, their yearly change in PSA was higher and at an average of 9 years prior to diagnosis, the PSA was increasing exponentially. Carter concludes that men with eventual metastatic disease harboured unrecognised disease at least 10 years prior to diagnosis.[86] Using figures from Gann,[87] he concluded that the lead time in diagnosis associated with PSA testing is 4–5 years.

Gleason scores and survival

Albertsen,[88] publishing in 1995, carried out competing risk analysis of men aged 55 to 74 years at diagnosis in a total of 767 men. Of 451 patients with T1 or T2 tumours treated with noncurative intent (immediate or delayed hormonal therapy only), he found that death from prostate cancer increased with Gleason score. This was a retrospective cohort study and did not measure PSA. He concluded that men with a Gleason score of 2–4 had a minimal risk of cancer-specific death from their disease within 15 years from diagnosis. Men with Gleason scores 5 and 6 had a modest risk of cancer-specific death but men with Gleason 7–10 have a high risk of cancer-specific death when treated conservatively.

In most men with localised CAP who present with moderately differentiated tumours, half will die from CAP if they live for 15 years.

The case for less aggressive treatment has also been made, and most persuasively by Chodak et al: they performed a pooled analysis of 6 non-randomised studies published since 1985 of 828 case records of men treated conservatively for clinically localised CAP.[89] The expected life expectancy was determined from standard life tables from the USA and Sweden. They verified that the proportional hazards model was appropriate and they then compared observed survival with Sweden's published life tables for the age of 70 using Cox regression and a similar method used to compare survival with US life tables. Disease-specific survival was calculated. Mortality at 10 years among men with grades 1 or 2 disease was 13% against 66% among men with grade 3 disease.

They concluded that watchful waiting was justified in men with grade 1 or 2 clinically localised disease, especially if their life expectancy was less than 10 years. They suggest that whether a higher rate of disease-free survival and metastasis-free survival is worth the risk of complications of aggressive therapy should be left to the patient to decide. They also conclude that in grade 3 cancers, neither radical surgery nor radiotherapy lowers the high rates of metastases and mortality seen with conservative treatments.

Metastases – suppressor genes

Initially, it was thought that metastases suppressor genes were merely a marker of metastatic ability. It is now believed that these genes regulate growth ability in secondaries. This is an exciting new development and current research is focusing particularly on the signalling pathways involved.[90]

It is accepted that hormonal treatment has a definite role in metastatic disease, but the timing of hormonal treatment in earlier disease is controversial. In general, in most cases, earlier treatment seems to produce better results.[91]

MANAGEMENT OF EARLY DISEASE

Diagnosis

Digital rectal examination can be of value if the examiner is experienced. Nodules may be felt, or a diffusely firm gland palpated, which can occasionally be rock hard. DRE alone misses a large number of early cancers.

A total of 75% of men with CAP will have abnormal PSAs.

The definitive diagnosis is made by biopsy carried out under TRUS. These biopsies are undertaken with prophylactic antibiotics such as a quinolone or co-amoxiclav given before and after biopsy.

A spring-assisted biopsy gun is used and biopsies taken of any hypoechoic areas, nodules felt per rectum (PR) or of six random areas of the prostate or more if felt necessary (some American centres suggest up to 12 biopsies).

Once the patient has been diagnosed as having early prostate cancer by a biopsy, then a full discussion must be had with the patient and preferably his spouse. He should already be aware of the implications of the diagnosis, but he will wish to discuss treatment in greater detail. The lack of randomised controlled trials (RCTs) makes giving advice difficult. The VAC-

URG trial is the only RCT of radical prostatectomy versus conservative management. No survival difference was demonstrated, but the study was underpowered and could not have demonstrated any expected small variance. Time to recurrence was reported, but long-term survival was not; although surgical patients fared better, the overall number of 97 was small.

If large trials are not available, we must examine the available data. Lu-Yao and Yao[92] reviewed the SEER (Surveillance, Epidemiology and End Results) database of 60,000 patients and reported treatment outcomes. Radical treatments were associated with better relative survival than an age-matched population, but disease-specific survival was unaffected by management policy.

More than one visit may be necessary to discuss the correct therapy for the patient, and second opinions should be offered freely.

Randomised trials are the only reliable way of minimising selection bias toward one treatment or another. Surgery may be biased to patients with more favourable disease and possibly with lower volume disease. Larger tumours which have surgery are more liable to be upstaged to T3.

The British Association of Urological Surgeons (BAUS) Working Party state that: 'there is good reason to question the current results of radical prostatectomy'. Even in the best departments, positive margin rates are obtained which would be unacceptable in other types of tumour.

The MRC trial of total prostatectomy versus radiotherapy versus no immediate treatment in early prostate cancer (PR06) was closed in September 1996 due to poor recruitment. Was it a victim of circumstance, untimely or a bad trial? The question was surely the most

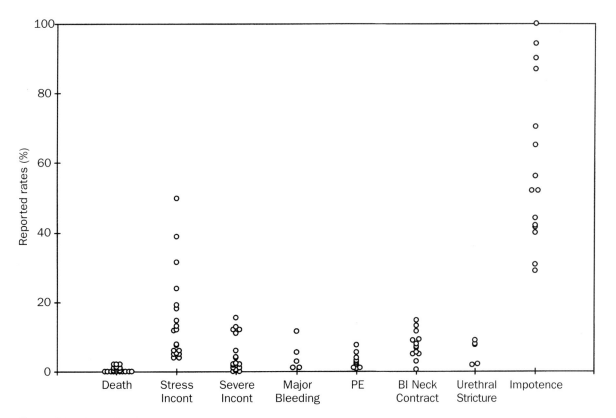

Figure 3.7 Complications: radical prostatectomy.

important to be posed by the current generation of urologists. Prostate cancer is increasing in incidence and there would scarcely have been a shortage of suitable patients.

Two similar trials are continuing to run: the prostate intervention versus observation trial (PIVOT) in North America and a similar Scandinavian study. Of the 10,000 new registrations with prostate cancer in the UK, 30% are within eligible stages (T1b/T1c/T2). It has been estimated that 40% of these patients (i.e. 1200) would be eligible.

Radical prostatectomy has a 10-year survival of 90% and disease-free survival of 75%. Nerve-sparing prostatectomy, as described by Walsh et al,[93] has reduced the morbidity and therefore increased the popularity of the operation. Incontinence rates are disputed, but are far from negligible. Impotence levels of 50% are widely quoted.

Morbidity and mortality of surgery

See Middleton (Figures 3.7 and 3.8).[94]

Radiotherapy

External beam radiotherapy has a disease-specific survival of 76% at 10 years in T1 and T2 carcinomas.

In, admittedly, small studies, the 10-year survival of patients without treatment with organ-confined prostate cancer has been reported at 85%, but these trials exclude patients with poorly differentiated cancers. The local progression rate in these untreated patients over 5 years was 50%. It can be difficult to diagnose cancer in patients and then to convince them that nothing need be done other than keeping it under surveillance.

Morbidity and mortality of radiotherapy
See Middleton (Figures 3.9 and 3.10).[94]

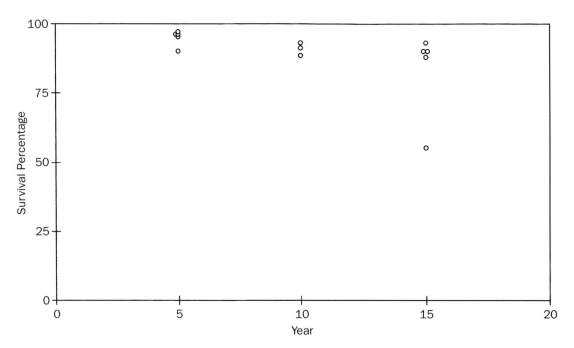

Figure 3.8 Disease-specific survival: radical prostatectomy.

Comparison of treatments

Referral to a specialist is often made for specific treatment and not for a choice. A surgical referral may be expected to lead to a surgical form of therapy. Many surgeons might find it difficult to admit to the uncertainty principle which governs RCTs and may find that any uncertainty leads to perceived erosion in patient confidence.

The number of surgical centres in the UK where radical prostatectomy is offered is still low, but increasing. Many surgeons may still be on the steep part of the learning curve for these operations and might not have wished early results to be subject to wider scrutiny. The 'no initial treatment option' may go against the therapeutic grain in specialists who are often overworked with respect to their US contemporaries and who may find it easier to institute immediate treatment.

To assess therapy, the natural history of the disease needs to be determined. In an age of evidence-based medicine (EBM), there is a hierarchy of evidence. The best situation is a meta-analysis of various large trials.

One way of advising patients in the absence of data from an RCT is to examine the data from the SEER study in USA.

SEER

Surveillance Epidemiology and End Results – A United States Central Cancer Registry on contract from the National Cancer Institute (NCI).

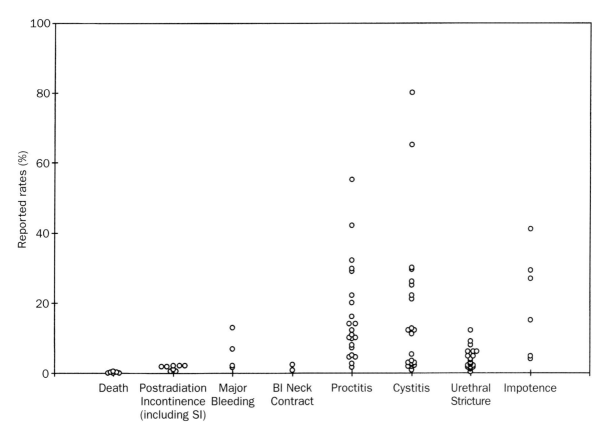

Figure 3.9 Complications: external beam radiotherapy.

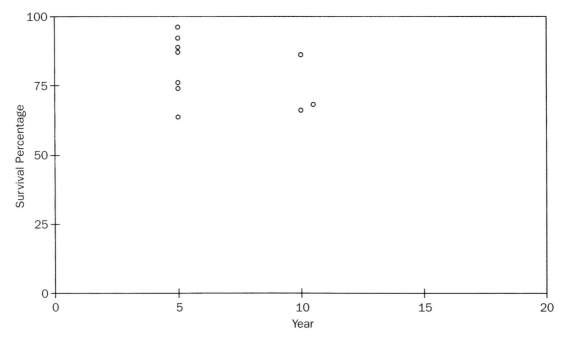

Figure 3.10 Disease-specific survival: external beam radiotherapy.

Lu-Yao & Yao[92] examined treatment outcomes from five districts in the USA in almost 60,000 patients. The relative outcomes are shown in Table 3.11.

There would appear to be a clear survival advantage in patients with grade 3 tumours treated with surgery and radiotherapy. The advantage is less marked in grade 2 tumours with both treatment modalities and only a marginal effect in grade 1 tumours. Surgery would appear to be clearly superior to radiotherapy in grade 3 tumours, but only marginally so in grade 2 tumours and to be of no increased benefit over radiotherapy in grade 1 tumours. Surgery removes all or the bulk of tumour, and it may be that this factor explains its clear superiority in this series in more active tumours. In Table 3.12 the treatments of external beam radiation therapy and radical prostatectomy are compared as regards complications.

D'Amico and his colleagues made an attempt at comparison based on biochemical failure, but of course survival analysis was not possible.[96]

Table 3.11 Outcome of treatment for early prostate cancer in 59,876 patients (SEER database). From Lu-Yao & Yao[92]

Grade and treatment	10-year relative survival (compared with age-matched cohort)
Grade I	
Prostatectomy	1.17
Radiotherapy	1.17
Surveillance	1.01
Grade II	
Prostatectomy	1.11
Radiotherapy	0.93
Surveillance	0.78
Grade III	
Prostatectomy	0.87
Radiotherapy	0.63
Surveillance	0.36

Table 3.12   Gastrointestinal or genitourinary complications and sexual dysfunction following definitive external beam radiation therapy or radical prostatectomy[95]

Symptom	Treatment	Baseline	12 months	24 months
At least mild tenderness or urgency during bowel movements	Surgery	3%	6%	2%
	Radiation therapy	2%	19%	18%
		$p > 0.05$	$p < 0.01$	$p < 0.01$
Urinary incontinence requiring pads (in last week)	Surgery	2%	35%	42%
	Radiation therapy	1%	5%	5%
		$p > 0.05$	$p < 0.001$	$p < 0.001$
Had no erections (in last 4 weeks)	Surgery	11%	75%	67%
	Radiation therapy	18%	33%	39%
		$p > 0.05$	$p < 0.001$	$p < 0.001$

Partin and his colleagues have derived a set of tables looking at risk at different levels of PSA (see appendix F).[97] Albertsen and his colleagues[98] used a technique of analysing competing risks for men aged 55–74 managed conservatively. They used a sample of 767 men managed conservatively by immediate or deferred hormone treatment from the Connecticut Tumor Registry with a minimum follow-up of 10 years. Their conclusions, mirrored by other authors, are as follows:

- Men with biopsy Gleason scores between 2 and 4 have a minimal risk of death from prostate cancer within the succeeding 15 years.
- Men with biopsy Gleason scores of 7–10 have a high risk of death from prostate cancer when treated conservatively (even up to age 74).
- Men with biopsy Gleason scores of 5–6 have a modest risk of death from prostate cancer. This risk increases slowly over a 15-year period.[100]

DETAILS OF THE TREATMENTS

Since the introduction of anatomical radical prostatectomy by Patrick Walsh, this surgical treatment has been increasingly popular.

The innovation which made it attractive was that using his technique it is possible to practice nerve sparing, which in theory spares the patient potency. Since many of these men are relatively young, particularly in the United States, it possessed an obvious attraction.

Pelvic lymphadenectomy is carried out at the time of operation and if lymph nodes are negative for the presence of tumour, the surgeon will proceed to radical removal of the prostate. This is normally carried out through the abdomen and is a major operation.

The results in skilled hands are excellent, but it does carry a mortality rate and a risk of severe bleeding. In many countries, blood is taken from the patient prior to surgery and then re-infused (autologous transfusion). There is a risk of incontinence, which may affect up to 25% of patients. It is essentially a form of stress incontinence and a small drip may be expressed when a patient bends over, e.g. when playing bowls.

Even in the best of hands, impotence can occur and, generally, the figure of 50% must be accepted.

The impotence can be treated subsequently, with sildenafil citrate (Viagra). This is a phosphodiesterase (PDE) inhibitor, which works principally on PDE5. Sexual arousal releases nitric oxide from nerve endings in the penis, which increases the production of cyclic guanosine monophosphate (GMP), a cyclic nucleotide, in vascular smooth muscle. PDE5 causes this nucleotide to be metabolised, and sildenafil inhibits this degradation, thus prolonging erection time and increasing turgidity. Disturbance of eyesight in some patients is believed to be due to action on PDE6, an isoenzyme found in eye tissue. Apomorphine in a sublingual dosage of 2 or 3mg may also be beneficial.

Survival in this group of patients is so long that it is necessary to assess results over a 10- or preferably a 15-year period. This is one of the reasons that we do not have conclusive evidence of the benefit of radical surgery.

Radical prostatectomy (OPCS CODE M6180, M611, 7B360)[99–101]

Hugh HamptonYoung first developed radical perineal prostatectomy in 1904 at the Johns Hopkins Hospital, Baltimore, Maryland. The retropubic approach was first introduced by Terence Millin. The side effects of the operation led to external beam radiotherapy becoming more popular and the surgical treatments became rare.

In the 1980s, Patrick Walsh, also at Johns Hopkins University, set out to identify the causes of failure of the surgical procedure. It was known that the procedure was associated with high blood loss, impotence and a significant incidence of urinary incontinence. He embarked on a series of studies. He identified the deep dorsal vein of the penis, running under Buck's fascia, and entering the urogenital diaphragm, dividing into the superficial branch, and the right and left lateral venous plexuses. The superficial branch lies outside the pelvic fascia. This fascia covers the lateral venous plexus.

Walsh devised a method of opening the endopelvic fascia, adjacent to the pelvic side wall, to avoid injury to the lateral venous plexus, division of the puboprostatic ligaments, while taking care not to injure the superficial branch of the dorsal vein, or enter the anterior prostatic fascia covering Santorini's plexus and the dorsal venous plexus and finally isolating the common trunk of the dorsal vein over the urethra, with a right-angled clamp, transecting this and controlling and avoiding most of the major bleeding.

Walsh then turned his attention to the autonomic innovation of the corpora cavernosa. The nerve supply emanates from the pudendal nerve and the pelvic plexus. The pudendal nerve provides autonomic supply to the corpora cavernosa and also the sensory supply to the skin. The exact location of the pelvic plexus and the branches to the corpora cavernosa were not known previously in man. He found that the capsular arteries and veins of a prostate served as scaffolding for the microscopic nerves and he demonstrated that the nerves were distributed, along with the capsular arteries and veins of the prostate, outside the capsule of the prostate. He demonstrated that the lateral and anterior pelvic fascia were reflected off the prostate. The neurovascular bundle is situated between the levator fascia and the prostate fascia.

Indications for radical prostatectomy

- Organ-confined prostate cancer
- The patient should have a life expectancy of at least 10 years
- The PSA should be <20.

Preoperative preparations
- Imaging – TRUS
- MR scan (optional)
- CT scan optional
- Blood tests
    haemoglobin
    full blood count
    urea and electrolytes
- Liver function tests, including isoenzymes for bone alkaline phosphatase
- Electrocardiography (ECG)
- Echocardiography, where indicated by significant cardiac disease.

If the PSA is less than 10, a bone scan is not necessary, although may be done to reassure the patient. If alkaline phosphatase is raised, a bone scan should be performed.

Cross-matching
A minimum of 6 units of packed cells are cross-matched.

Heparin
It is customary to give the patient 5000 units of heparin subcutaneously twice daily preoperatively and until the patient is ambulant.

Theatre allocation
An operating time of at least 4 hours is commonly booked. Ideally, two assistants must be free, at least one of whom is experienced.

Consent
Radical prostatectomy implies removal of the prostate and the iliac and the lymph nodes between the obturator neurovascular bundle and the external iliac vein. Operative and perioperative risks of bleeding, pain and infection must be addressed. Fatigue in the medium term is best mentioned, and the risks and rates of incontinence and impotence must be discussed.

Admission
The patient is generally brought into the ward 1 day prior to surgery and patch-tested for iodine. Subcutaneous heparin is started on the same day and until the patient is mobilised, and compression (anti-thrombo-embolic stockings, TED) applied. Where the patient is unfit, it is also prudent to ensure that there is an intensive therapy unit (ITU) bed available.

Instruments
• Laparotomy crate – major general set
• Ring retractor – Bookwalter™ or Munster™
• Bipolar diathermy
• Wallace drain introducer
• MacDougall's right- and left-angle clamps
• Headlight.

Long instruments
Double-action needle holder.

Patient position
In the USA, the operation is performed under spinal anaesthesia, but in the UK the operation is performed under general anaesthesia, with muscle relaxation and preoperative preparation.

Surgery is deferred for 6–8 weeks after needle biopsy of the prostate and 12 weeks after TURP.

In certain circumstances, the patient may be asked to donate blood for autologous transfusion.

The patient is placed in the supine position, with the table broken at the umbilicus. The table is then tilted into a Trendelenburg position. A 16-French (16F) Foley catheter is passed into the bladder and inflated with 30 ml of saline. The catheter is then placed on free drainage. A midline extraperitoneal lower abdominal incision is made from the pubis to the umbilicus. The rectus muscles are divided.

The pelvic lymph nodes are dissected and the lymphatics over the external iliac artery are preserved, but the lymph nodes are removed down the pelvic side wall and towards the femoral canal.

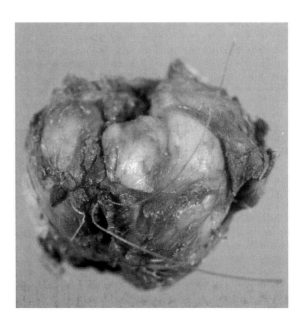

Figure 3.11 Radical prostatectomy specimen.

An incision is made in the endopelvic fascia, lateral enough to avoid damaging the veins of Santorini's plexus. The puboprostatic ligaments are transected and then the dorsal vein complex isolated and divided using the MacDougall right-angle clamps. The anterior two-thirds of the urethra is divided without damaging the Foley catheter. Dissolvable sutures may be placed in a distal urethral segment. The catheter balloon is deflated and the posterior area of urethra is divided. Walsh explains this technique in great detail.

The neurovascular bundles are preserved at the apex. Lateral pedicles are divided usually in two portions. Buck's fascia is divided near the tip of the seminal vesicles and the vesicles can be dissected at this stage.

Once the prostate is removed, the bladder neck is reconstituted using interrupted dissolvable 2/0 sutures. Taking the mucosa in these sutures cuts down on haematuria.

A further Foley catheter is inserted *per urethram* and 3/0 sutures are placed on the distal urethra and then completed by passing them through the bladder and its mucosa.

The catheter is introduced through the bladder neck, into the bladder, and thereafter the sutures are tied. The bladder is irrigated to ensure that no clots have built up.

Closure
The wound is closed in layers, with two suction drains with polydioxanone polyfilament absorbable sutures (ETHICON).

Postoperative care
The patient's vital signs are monitored and urine output charted. A small degree of haematuria is expected. The drains are removed when they stop draining. The specimen is sent for pathological examination using carefully devised sectioning techniques.[102]

Specific complications – early
Mortality 0.2%.

Intraoperative complications
- Bleeding
- Obturator nerve injury
- Rectal injury.

Postoperative complications – early
- Delayed bleeding
- Penile oedema/bruising
- Lymphocele.

Postoperative complications – late
- Incontinence
- Impotence.

Erectile dysfunction (ED)
The Massachusetts Male Aging Study gives one of the best indications of erectile dysfunction and its increase with ageing. It is a surprise to discover that even amongst 40-year-old men, only 60% would have erections. The data from 70-year-old men showed that 30% of men were potent at age 70 and the rate of complete impotence increased threefold to 15%.[104] It is important that changes in potency are related to preoperative levels.

Margin positivity
About 50% of men with positive margins progress after surgery. The following section looks at technical failures. There is an overall positive margin rate of between 11 and 15%, and PSA control of less than 1 ng/ml in between 90 and 95% of cases. Continence rates vary between 37 and 60% at 1 month and between 68 and 95% at 9 months. It is said to take at least 50 cases for an experienced surgeon to learn the technique. At present, this technique, although of interest, raises questions as to how exportable it is outside of specialist centres.[105–107]

Perineal prostatectomy

A number of centres practice radical perineal prostatectomy. The advantage of this technique is lower blood loss. It is a matter of debate as to whether the nerve sparing is equivalent to an open operation.

Laparoscopic radical prostatectomy

At present, this technique remains confined to a few centres and we need further information, both about the safety of cancer control and perioperative morbidity.

Radiotherapy

External beam radiotherapy for early prostate cancer has its advocates. The absence of RCTs makes comparison with other treatments difficult. Because it may be perceived as less traumatic for the patient, the treated population tends to be older, which affects direct comparison with surgical options.

Although staging is carried out by CT scanning, patients receiving radiotherapy do not usually have pathological lymph node staging, which will have the net effect of including more patients with more advanced stage of disease than those reported in surgical series. PSA testing has reduced this bias.

Radiotherapy works by disrupting DNA in the tumour, but it may take many months or even several years for all the cancer cells to be disrupted sufficiently. It is known from post-treatment biopsy studies that apparently active cancer cells can be found in the prostate for several years and this correlates with an increased risk of death from prostate cancer. Normal glands atrophy, and fibrosis is observed. The number and size of malignant glands decrease and their nuclei become irregular. It is disputed if Gleason grading is appropriate after radiotherapy.

CT planning is carried out before treatment in a supine position with a full bladder (Figure 3.12). The target volume is the prostate plus a margin of 1.5–2 cm. The rectum receives a significant dose of radiation, and this is the cause of subsequent proctitis. Coexisting diseases of the bowel such as inflammatory bowel disease is a contraindication.

The treatments are given in fractions, usually using one anterior and two posterior fields using a high-energy linear accelerator. Tattoo marks are placed in the patient's skin to ensure correct alignment at each session.

The total dose is between 55 and 64 Gy in the UK but is considerably higher in the USA, in fractions of 2–2.75 Gy/day. Total treatment time is over a period of 7 weeks.

Side effects are dose-related and include bladder and bowel symptoms, usually frequency proctitis and diarrhoea. Late side effects can emerge in the bladder, bowel and urethra between 6 months and 2 years after treatment. Major complications occur in 2–3% of reported series. Steroid enemata can be efficacious in treatment.

Radiotherapy may have poorer results if the pretreatment PSA is greater than 15 ng/ml. The PSA nadir should be less than 1 ng/ml post-treatment. The addition of hormonal treatment to radiotherapy appears to increase response rates (see below).

Efficacy – biopsy following radiotherapy for early prostate cancer

Post-radiotherapy biopsies may show residual tumour in anything between 18 and 65% of cases.[108–111]

Only a minority of patients who have had radiotherapy have post-radiation biopsies. The reasons for the differences in rates include:

1. serum PSA at the time of biopsy
2. stage and grade of original tumour
3. radiotherapy technique and dose
4. time interval since radiotherapy
5. biopsy technique and number of cores
6. the experience of the pathologist and the use of appropriate immunohistochemical stains.[112]

Most treatment biopsies appear to vary with post-treatment PSA levels.

It can be difficult to determine which of the cells are fatally damaged by radiation. Proliferation markers, such as PCNA (proliferative cell nuclear androgen) and MIB1 can be used. Unfortunately, PCNA is affected by how long the tissues have been fixed and stains normally proliferating cells and also those that are being repaired, as a consequence of radiation damage.

Crook and his colleagues suggested a

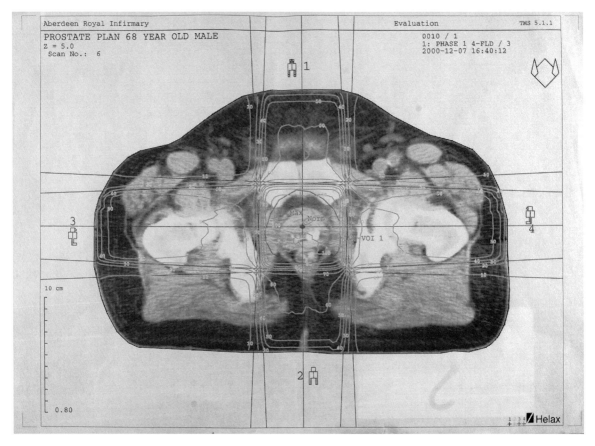

Figure 3.12 Prostate radiotherapy plan.

grading scheme for cytoplastic and nuclear radiation effects in cells and evaluated cancer-free survival with their pathological evaluations (Table 3.13).[112–115]

Improving the results with hormonal treatment
Bolla et al[116] published a Phase III randomised trial of 415 patients, initiated by the European Organization for Research and Treatment of Cancer (EORTC) to compare adjuvant hormone therapy, using goserelin, given at the onset of radiotherapy, with radiotherapy alone. In both treatment arms, 50 Gy was given to the pelvis over 5 weeks, with a further 20 Gy boost to the prostate over 2 weeks. Goserelin was administered 4 weekly for 3 years and cyproterone acetate was given for the first month of treat-

ment. On analysis, 385 patients were evaluable, with a median follow-up of 33 months. Overall survival rates of 78% for adjuvant hormone therapy, in addition to radiotherapy, compared favourably with an overall survival rate of 56% for radiotherapy alone. This suggests that adjuvant hormonal therapy treatment from the onset of external irradiation improves local control and survival.

The cytoreductive effect of LH RH agonists in bulky disease was determined in trial RTOG 86–10. This involved 471 patients. LH RH treatment was given 2 months before and 2 months during definitive irradiation, compared with patients in the standard arm receiving immediate radiation only. There was an improvement in clinical disease-free survival in the LH

RH group of 61% versus 43% and also in survival with a PSA level of less than 4 ng/ml (46% versus 26%).[116,117]

The value of a joint consultation with a radiotherapist and a surgeon is that these issues can be brought to the patient's attention and the treatment which is thought to be best for the patient can be selected, after full and frank discussion.

Conformal radiotherapy

Conventional delivery of the radiotherapy beam is in the shape of a cube. Using multileaf collimators, software programs allow the beam shape to be adjusted to spare normal tissues, and this new technique is believed to reduce

late damage to bowel. More recent linear accelerators have these modifications and allow ever more sophisticated planning and delivery of treatment.

Brachytherapy in prostate cancer

Interstitial brachytherapy of the prostate began in 1910, when Pasteau and Degrais used radium needles inserted through the perineum into the prostate. This was done by guiding the needles, with fingers in the rectum. Subsequently, there have been attempts made to use radioactive substances implanted during open operation. In 1972, Whitmore used iodine 125 seed implantation through an open operation when he was carrying out pelvic lymph node dissection.

The invention of ultrasound allowed for identification of the areas of cancer, and in 1981 Holm in Denmark introduced ultrasound-guided seed implantation of abdominal tumours and developed a technique for needle placement in the prostate guided by TRUS.

In the 1980s, Ragde, working in Seattle refined the technique and, with Blasko, treated many patients.

Holm & Gammelgaard[118] described in 1981 the technique of TRUS with a template guidance system, to allow accurate positioning of needles within the prostate. Although this was first used for biopsy, it was soon realised that this could be used to guide radioactive sources into specific areas in the prostate and could be done in real time, using dynamic ultrasound. This led to the establishment of the modern technique of brachytherapy. It must be appreciated that the technique is a two-stage procedure. The first stage is to use TRUS to measure the prostatic volume and to use the data obtained to plan the number and positioning of a radioactive source, in an attempt to deliver a homogeneous dose of radiation to the prostate.

The second stage involves the sources being inserted into the replanned position, using a template.

At present, these needles are inserted through the perineal skin, as a closed procedure.

Table 3.13 Serious complications of radiation therapy in cancer of the prostate. Summary of complications in 658 patients[112]

Symptoms	Per cent
Bowel symptoms	
Anal stricture	0.3
Rectal stricture	0.1
Anal fissure	0.1
Small bowel obstruction	0.5
Urinary symptoms	
Urethral stricture	3.0
Haematuria	0.6
Urinary incontinence	0.6
Ureteral stricture	0.1
Vesicosigmoid fistula	0.1
Rectovesical fistula	0.1
Ureteral stricture	0.3
Other	
Severe oedema	1.0
Impotence	18 (this was measured against patients who were potent at the time of radiation therapy)[115]

Ultrasound is favoured over CT imaging, since the latter can overestimate the prostate volume. It is important, as with all radiotherapy, to minimise the dose nearest the rectal wall, since this is likely to produce radiation proctitis. Software programs determine the total radiation dose. Implants can be either removed or permanent.

Removable implants

The removable implants can be either continuous low-dose rate, using low-activity iridium wire, or high-dose rate implant. These removable implants can not be tolerated for more than a day or two and, with most of these techniques, an additional boost of fractionated external beam radiation is given.

Permanent implants

Permanent implants are the most common type of energy source. The seeds are left within the prostate and they deliver radiation over a period of weeks or months. Iodine 125 has a half-life of 60 days and it is usual to prescribe a minimum peripheral dose of 160 Gy to a volume which includes the prostate capsule plus a 2 or 3 mm margin. Palladium, which is commonly used in the USA, has a half-life of 17 days and can occasionally be used for tumours with a higher Gleason score.

Iodine 125 has an energy of 27–35 kV, which means that there is little penetration into tissues. The inverse square law of radiation states that the dose is inversely proportional to the square of the distance from the source and, in the example of iodine, less than 50% of the minimal peripheral dose is delivered within a few millimetres of the source. Theoretically, this should have an advantage in terms of damage to adjacent structures such as the rectum and the nerves, which run alongside the prostate. The disadvantage is that disease extending more than 3 or 4 mm outside the prostate capsule will not be irradiated.

The technique requires an experienced team and there should be, at a minimum, a clinical oncologist, support staff, a radiologist with expertise in performing ultrasound techniques, an anaesthetist and a nurse coordinator who carries out counselling, coordinating and timing of implants, instruction of replacement of seeds, education of staff and care of patients, etc.[119]

Selection criteria

The selection criteria are that:

- the patient has a biopsy confirming adenocarcinoma of the prostate
- the disease must be confined within the prostate capsule, mainly T1 to T2C, as confirmed by TRUS and/or endorectal MR scanning
- there must be no evidence of metastatic disease
- the patient's life expectancy must be greater than 10 years
- the volume of the prostate should be less than 50 ml
- PSA should be less than 50
- there should be an absence of severe urinary obstruction, and there should be no severe pubic arch interference.

If there is thought to be extracapsular involvement, staging biopsies may be performed under ultrasound control.

There is controversy about the role of LH RH analogues and/or androgen blockers, which may be given for 3 months prior to brachytherapy to reduce the volume of prostate. These may be given where waiting lists for treatment are long.

If the patient has had a TURP, the results of brachytherapy are less predictable and many centres would not undertake brachytherapy where a TURP has been carried out. Patients who have had a TURP have a high risk of developing incontinence.[119]

Morbidity and mortality (Figures 3.13 and 3.14)

Patients can develop obstructive and irritative urinary symptoms following prostate brachytherapy. In larger series, between 4 and 8% of patients require minor surgical procedures such as catheterisation or cystoscopy in the post-treatment phase.

Proctitis occurs in less than 2% of patients

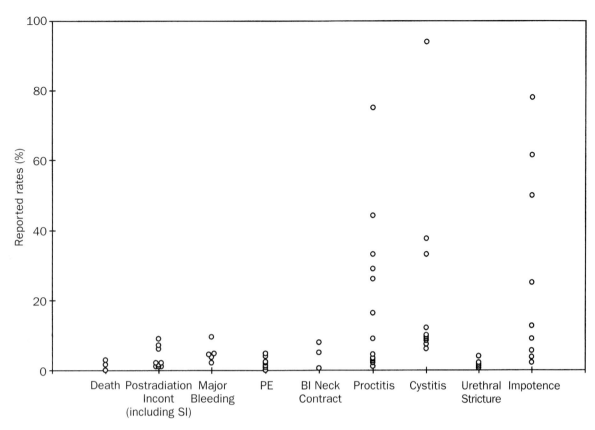

Figure 3.13 Complications: brachytherapy (interstitial radiotherapy).

receiving seed implants as the sole treatment. Incontinence occurs in up to 1% of patients where there has been no previous TURP.

Where a TURP has been performed, the incontinence rate is said to be up to 50%, although this figure may be debated. The advocates of brachytherapy emphasise the advantages of convenience, cost, low morbidity and efficacy. Few studies of mortality are available (Figure 3.14).

Results
PSA control at 2–5 years for the different series ranges from 76 to 98%. Naturally, pretreatment factors such as baseline PSA, Gleason score and clinical stage are strong predictors of clinical outcome.

For higher-risk localised prostate cancers, for Gleason scores greater than or equal to 7, and with a high initial PSA, some centres combine external beam radiation with radioactive seed implants.[120–122]

Results from Blasko and his colleagues[121,122] indicate that an at least 80% pathologically confirmed local control rate, following interstitial brachytherapy, is obtained in early prostate cancer. It is known that patients with indeterminate biopsies may convert being negative over time, the effect on the cells being cumulative; usually the initial radiation effect will have disappeared. Follow-up can also be estimated using PSA levels. Actuarial clinical control of disease is 83%, but biochemical disease-free survival reports and literature are immature

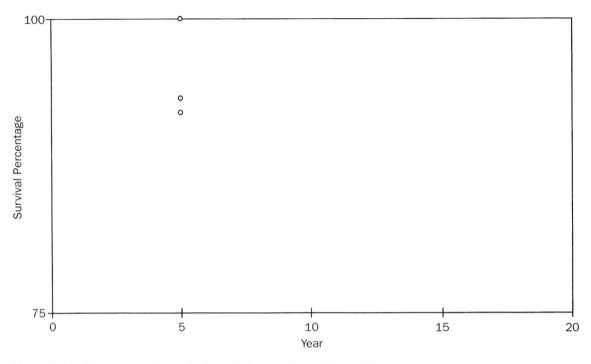

Figure 3.14 Disease-specific survival: brachytherapy (interstitial radiotherapy).

and are difficult at present to compare to the results obtained by radical prostatectomy or standard radiation therapy.

The technique for iodine 125 seed implantation (See Figure 3.15)

1. The patient's cancer is confirmed by the DRE, PSA and histology.
2. TRUS is used to give volume study of the prostate gland. This provides the treatment dosage model.
3. Pre-implant dosimetry is used to determine the number of seeds, their location and activity. The seeds are then ordered for the implant, with a lead to order time of approximately 4 weeks.
4. The patient has a general anaesthetic and is placed in the dorsal-lithotomy position.
5. The seeds are implanted, in accordance with the seed plan.
6. Postoperative care may also involve insertion of a Foley catheter. Those patients go home the same day.
7. Follow-up procedures – checking of the position and dosimetry of the seeds, by a CT scan. It is important that the dose distribution of the seeds is determined to estimate post-implant dosimetry. This involves reconstruction from simulator films, using either plain films or a CT reconstruction.

Cryotherapy

Cryotherapy has been used in the prostate for many years, but recently the ability to monitor temperature and prevent the urethra from being damaged by the use of warming catheters has given the modality a new lease of life. Up to eight cryogenic probes are inserted through the perineum under ultrasound-guided control. A cooling agent such as argon or liquid nitrogen is circulated through the probes, which reduces the tissue temperature to −40°C. This is seen as an ice ball and, since it forms so rapidly, the cell membranes are disrupted, killing the cells in

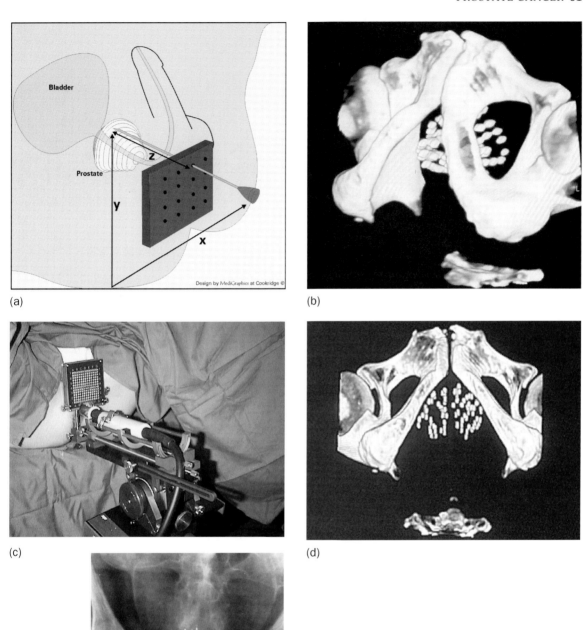

Figure 3.15 (a) Schematic representation of prostate implant. (b) Diagram of seed placement in relation to pelvic bones. (c) TRUS probe in situ and GMD in place prior to seed placement. (d) Relationship of seeds to pubic arch. (e) Post-implantation seed positions.

the vicinity. Several freeze–thaw cycles are carried out under general anaesthetic.

Early 5-year data suggest that the technique is safe, and is effective in reducing PSA. Higher morbidity rates are seen in patients who have had a prior TURP or radiation therapy. It has a high rate of impotence.[123,124]

Other unproven treatments

High-intensity focussed ultrasound and radiofrequency energy have been used to deliver cytotoxic levels of energy to tumour tissue, but there is no evidence to demonstrate the superiority of these techniques in terms of efficacy.

The role of hormonal therapy in early prostate cancer has yet to be established. There are a number of studies looking at the effect of Casodex (bicalutamide), an anti-androgen, for the long-term management of these patients.

Watchful waiting

Patients may elect to have no treatment at all at an early stage of their disease. There are many patients for whom this is a sensible option, particularly if they are unwell from coexisting medical conditions.

Radiation therapy is often used as adjuvant of salvage therapy in men with persistent recurring PSA levels after surgery. It is of course only of use in local recurrence.[125]

Hormonal therapy after failure of local treatment

Treatment of patients who have failed local therapy is controversial. Schulman and colleagues found only one randomised study by Messing, looking at adjuvant hormonal therapy in patients with lymph node positive disease found at the time of surgery. Ninety-eight patients were randomised to receive adjuvant hormonal therapy or observation. Seven of the 47 patients treated with immediate hormonal therapy, either goserelin or bilateral orchidectomy, had died at follow-up (median 7 years), compared with 18 of 51 patients in the observation group. This difference is statistically highly significant.[125,126]

Prayer-Galetti and his colleagues randomised 201 patients with stage C prostate cancer, who were treated with radical prostatectomy to receive either no treatment or treatment with goserelin over 28 days, beginning 15 days after surgery. Disease-free survival was significantly longer with patients treated with hormonal therapy, but this group included a disproportionate number of patients with low-to-moderate Gleason scores and no seminal vesicle involvement.[125,126]

Longer follow-up is necessary.

Treatment failure after primary radiotherapy

Prostatic biopsy has been used in assessing treatment failure, but a PSA nadir may be more effective in judging failure. There is debate as to the level of nadir which can be accepted as indicating a good prognosis.[102,103,127,128]

Salvage surgery following failed radiotherapy treatment

The main problem with this group of patients is that of surgical complication, such as urinary incontinence and blood loss. Incontinence rates can be very high and salvage surgery is rarely practised in the UK. Surprisingly, a disease-free survival of 47% has been reported in one study.[129,130]

Hormonal therapy after local curative treatment failure

Much of the evidence for hormonal treatment has been gathered from studies such as the Medical Research Council (MRC) study of immediate versus deferred hormone therapy.[131] The timing of treatment in this group of patients is still dubious and the results of the studies are awaited. It may be at present that in older men with low-risk disease, with low-volume prostate cancer, who harbour well-differentiated tumours, deferred treatment may be the best option in this group.[130]

Margin positive disease prevention

Attempts have been made to improve surgical margins by downsizing, downstaging and downgrading of tumours by preoperative treatment with anti-androgens or an LH RH agonist.[130] Not surprisingly, this treatment reduces the positive margin rate, but no improvement in survival has been demonstrated. It is possible that this downstaging has been a way of qualifying patients for operation rather than improving their biological chances of cure. It is known that pretreatment using androgen deprivation therapy reduces the PSA nadir by 14% within 3 months and by 84% at 8 months.[103]

MANAGEMENT OF ADVANCED DISEASE

> MRC – Immediate versus deferred treatment for advanced prostate cancer – Why treat?

This question appears redundant now but, at the time of its launch, many urologists in the UK were convinced that treatment was often more dangerous than no treatment; this was the era of oestrogens, sometimes in very high dosage.

MRC study

This was a large multicentre trial, that ran from 1985 to 1993. Patients with histologically proven cancer of the prostate for whom there was genuine doubt as to whether hormone treatment was immediately required were randomised either to immediate hormone treatment or to delay treatment until specific indication for hormonal treatment arose.[132]

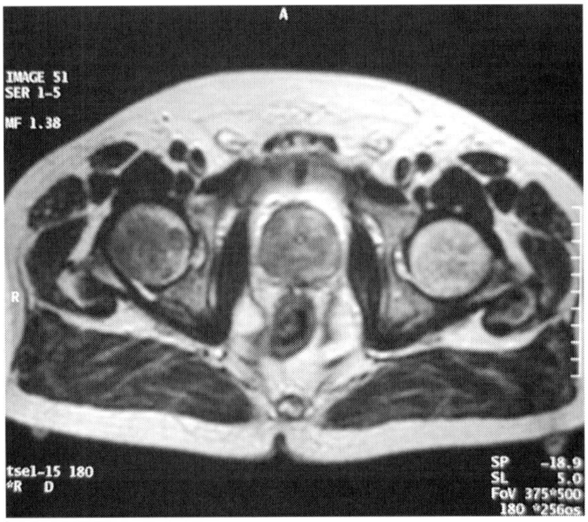

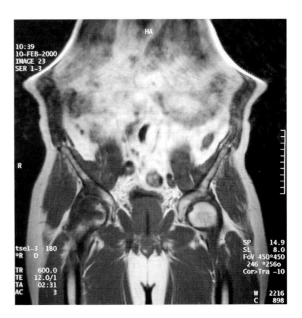

Figure 3.16 Axial T2 MR image of pelvis showing right-sided primary prostatic tumour and femoral head metastasis.

Figure 3.17 Coronal T1 MR image of pelvis in same patient showing skeletal metastases in right femoral head and acetabulum from primary prostate.

The results indicated that there was a clear reduction of side complications in patients who received immediate treatment. This was judged by a lower number of spinal cord collapses and channel TURPs required for prostatic obstruction.

This study was important because it focussed the attention of British urologists on the long-term follow-up of patients. Previously, it had often been concluded that the patients would die from other diseases than their prostate cancer. It was a surprise to many to find that a lot of these elderly men were in fact dying from their prostate cancer. This focussed interest in prostate cancer in the UK in a way that no other previous study had done.

It must be remembered that the study was carried out against a background of traditional stilboestrol treatment, which was known to have a high cardiovascular complication rate, despite its undoubted efficacy. Major complications found in this study are listed in Table 3.14.

Patients who present with disease which has escaped from the prostatic capsule or have a high burden of disease due to secondaries in the bone should first be staged by bone scanning.

The treatment of advanced disease is essentially hormonal.

Androgen deficiency

Androgen deficiency in the ageing male is a gradual event. It has effects on bone metabolism, muscular and adipose tissue, sleep patterns, mood, intellectual activities and psychological and physical well-being.[133]

Oestrogens

These were the main treatment used in the early days of treatment. The dose of oestrogen has been progressively lowered due to cardiovascular side effects. When response occurs, it is usually long-lasting and durable, but the high incidence of side effects has meant that the drug is no longer recommended as first-line therapy. It may be employed for hormonally escaped prostate cancer. It is now a cheap drug and does have a role in developing countries, but the low cost of bilateral orchiectomy makes this a preferred treatment for many patients.[134,135]

The treatment options are now considered.

Bilateral orchiectomy

Surgical castration may be by removal of the entire testicle or by using a technique called subcapsular orchiectomy where the capsule of the testicle is left intact, thus giving an appearance of a testicle within the scrotum. Both methods are effective in producing a castrate level of androgens.[136–138]

In men with prostate cancer, this remains an effective technique and is practised extensively worldwide. It is still considered the 'gold standard' of hormonal treatment. Although the surgical treatment is initially expensive, it avoids the need for subsequent medication and for many patients it is an appropriate and cost-effective treatment.[139]

Anti-androgens

Anti-androgens are divided into two groups: the pure anti-androgens and those with steroidal components.

Steroidal anti-androgens
Cyproterone acetate is a steroidal anti-androgen, having actions both against androgen and progestogens. Because of its high side-effect profile, cyproterone acetate has been restricted to pretreating patients prior to LH RH releasing analogues.

Pure anti-androgens
The main example of this type of drug has been flutamide. Flutamide is a pure anti-androgen and, unfortunately, has quite a number of side effects. It does, however, have the benefit of a lower rate of impotence, but it is prudent to discuss with the patient that there may be a trade

Table 3.14   Major complications found in MRC study

Complication	Immediate (n = 469)	Deferred (n = 465)
Pathological fracture		
M0	3	6
Mx	1	4
M1	7	11
Total	11	21
Cord compression		
M0	3	3
Mx	1	6
M1	5	14
Total	9	23
Ureteric obstructions		
M0	22	28
Mx	1	12
M1	10	15
Total	33	55
Extraskeletal metastases		
M0	17	26
Mx	7	9
M1	13	20
Total	37	55

off against survival. There are no large studies to show its equivalence to other treatments.[144,145]

It was originally used as a monotherapy for advanced prostate cancer, but became less popular with time. It has recently enjoyed an increase in usage as part of maximal androgen blockade (MAB).

LH RH analogues

LH RH releasing analogues, given by injection either monthly or 3-monthly, have become extremely popular for obvious reasons. The side-effect profile is low and the patient avoids the need for taking tablets daily and thus being reminded of his disease.[140–143]

Bicalutamide

Recently licensed as monotherapy in the UK, bicalutamide was originally used as one com-

ponent of MAB, along with an LH RH analogue.[143]

Androgen deprivation strategies are shown in Table 3.15.

Effects of anti-androgen treatments

Schroder and his EORTC colleagues examined sexual function after flutamide and other anti-androgens.[145] They make the important point that diagnosis of prostate cancer seems in itself to have considerable impact on libido and therefore on sexual function. In a small number of patients, sexual recovery can occur when the patient was impotent prior to treatment.

In general, however, sexual function with flutamide treatment was higher in patients on cyproterone acetate. However, the differences did not reach statistical significance, despite the sample of 294 men.[145]

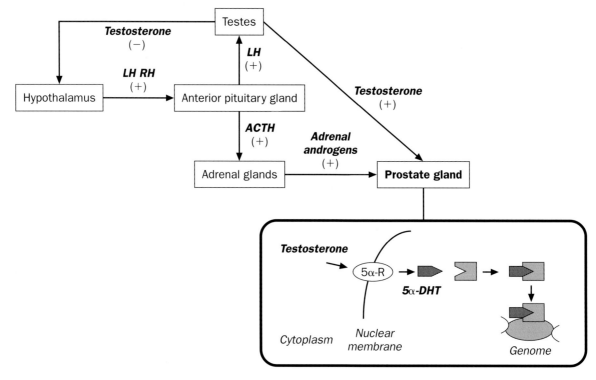

Figure 3.18 Regulation of androgens and their mechanism of action in the prostate gland. LH RH = luteinising hormone-releasing hormone, LH = luteinising hormone, ACTH = adrenocorticotropic hormone, 5α-R = 5α-reductase, 5α-DHT = 5α-dihydrotestosterone, + = activation, − = inhibition.

Fatigue in patients with prostate cancer

Stone and his colleagues carried out a study examining fatigue in 62 patients and found that fatigue is common and under-recognised as a side effect of hormone therapy. This appeared to be independent of anaemia and was not related to nausea or vomiting.[146]

Summary of side effects of treatments

Orchiectomy
- Hot flushes
- Gynaecomastia
- Reduced libido
- Impotence
- ?Psychological impact of losing testes.

LH RH analogue: e.g. leuprorelin, goserelin, buserelin, triptorelin
- Hot flushes
- Gynaecomastia
- Reduced libido
- Impotence
- Risk of 'flare' reaction on starting treatment.

Nonsteroidal anti-androgens: e.g. flutamide, bicalutamide
- Painful gynaecomastia
- Diarrhoea
- Indigestion
- Hepatotoxicity.

Steroidal anti-androgens: e.g. cyproterone acetate
- Fluid retention
- Lethargy

Table 3.15   Androgen deprivation strategies

Therapy	Advantages	Disadvantages
Orchiectomy	Gold standard for treatment of advanced prostate cancer	Definitive castration
	Relatively simple operation	Associated psychological trauma
	Ablation of testicular source of testosterone	Loss of sexual potency
	Rapid tumour response	Hot flushes
		Reduced muscle mass and energy
		Anaemia and osteoporosis
		Adrenal androgens unaffected
Diethylstilboestrol	Ablation of testicular source of testosterone	Loss of sexual potency
		Gynaecomastia
		Sometimes fatal cardiovascular side effects
		Reduced immune response
		Adrenal androgens unaffected
LH RH[a] analogues:	More acceptable to patients than orchiectomy	Transient 'flare' of symptoms during first week of therapy
goserelin	Reversible medical castration	Loss of sexual potency
leuprolide	Ablation of testicular source of testosterone	Hot flushes
triptorelin		Reduced muscle mass and energy
		Anaemia and osteoporosis
		Adrenal androgens unaffected
Steroidal anti-androgens:	Competitive inhibition of androgens from testes and adrenal glands	Central inhibitory effect
cyproterone acetate		Progestogenic activity
megestrol acetate		Loss of sexual potency
		Fluid retention, thrombophlebitis and cardiovascular side effects
Nonsteroidal anti-androgens	Competitive inhibition of androgens from testes and adrenal glands	Gynaecomastia and breast pain
flutamide		Diarrhoea (especially flutamide)
nilutamide	Sexual potency preserved	Hepatotoxicity
bicalutamide	Good tolerability (especially bicalutamide)	Visual disturbances, respiratory disturbances and alcohol intolerance (nilutamide only)
	Once-daily dosing regimen (nilutamide and bicalutamide)	

[a]LH RH = luteinising hormone-releasing hormone.

- Reduced libido
- Hepatotoxicity.

Oestrogens: e.g. stilboestrol
- Thromboembolic risk
- Fluid retention
- Gynaecomastia
- Reduced libido
- Impotence.

Paraneoplastic syndromes

There are a number of paraneoplastic syndromes associated with prostate cancer:

- Inappropriate antidiuretic hormone secretion
- Cushing's syndrome
- hypercalcaemia
- hypophosphataemia
- human chorionic gonadotropin (HCG)
- bleeding diathesis and coagulation disorders
- neuromuscular
- dermatomyositis.

Maximal androgen blockade (MAB)

It had long been realised that the testicles produce 90% of androgens but the remaining 10% came from the adrenals. Extensive attempts were made to combine androgen blockade by reducing testicular androgens and blocking the remaining adrenal androgens by anti-androgen therapy. These trials took up much of the 1990s and continue to provoke debate. Despite the mammoth number of patients, in excess of 10,000, there has been little evidence of superiority. The meta-analyses of these trials have not demonstrated anything other than small effects. Patients who are younger and who have a small disease burden are believed to benefit most but, for most patients, the effects on survival are negligible, and purchased at the expense of increased side effects.[147–150]

Intermittent hormone therapy

In the quest for control of advanced prostate cancer, hormonal treatment has been tried from almost every angle. Possibly because some patients have decided to stop their treatment for several months, the concept of intermittent treatment has become more popular.[151,152] The patient whose disease is in abeyance may stop his treatment while the PSA is observed. There have been no large studies to ascertain whether this is a safe option, but there is no doubt that there are many patients who seem to keep their PSA at a low level, in the absence of treatment, for periods as long as 6 months. This can be a reasonable option, although there has been concern that this will 'let the genie out of the bottle'. In practice, few patients seem to have done badly with this regimen. It is imperative that the PSA is monitored closely, at monthly or 2-monthly intervals and that treatment be resumed on any significant increase of the PSA level. This sequence may be followed on a number of occasions, but does require a patient who is both well motivated and well informed.

Patients will respond for about 2 years on any form of hormonal treatment. At this point, the patients who are seen at regular intervals often begin to show an increase in their PSA. This precedes the advent of symptoms and, at that stage, the physician normally keeps these patients under review and may wish to enter them into a clinical trial.

MANAGEMENT OF COMPLICATIONS OF ADVANCED DISEASE

Ureteric obstruction. Endoscopic insertion of a J–J stent into the ureter (M2920, M292, 7B1A1)

The patient is placed in the lithotomy position and a standard cystoscopy is undertaken, using an image intensifier.

A flexible tipped guidewire is inserted through the channel in the cystoscope. This is introduced into the ureteric orifice and pushed under screening control into the pelvis of the

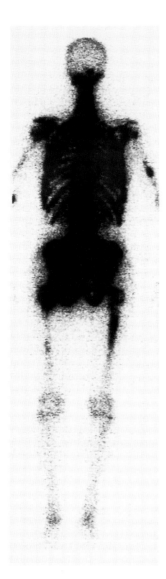

Figure 3.19 Isotope bone scan showing 'superscan' appearance from extensive metastases from primary prostate cancer.

the guidewire and gently pushed through the cystoscope. It is wise to check in advance that the gauge of the stent will be accommodated by the channel gauge of the cystoscope.

It can be introduced alongside the cystoscope, but this creates a tight area at the bladder neck and can lead to difficulties later. Once the stent is pushed along the guidewire, a pusher is then introduced onto the guidewire and this is used to push the stent into the ureter.

It is wise to keep a note of the gradations or markers on the stent, to ensure that it is not pushed too far.

Once the final 2–3 cm are seen entering the bladder, it is sensible to re-screen at this point to ensure that the stent is within the kidney. It is now necessary to ask the assistant to withdraw the guidewire, keeping a hand on the pusher. The J end of the stent will then curl up within the bladder.

It is good practice to keep a note of the details of the stent and its batch number, etc. This should be placed on the operation note, in the patient record.

Many units keep an independent note of stents which are inserted, to ensure that they are not left in inadvertently.

If retrograde placement of stent is impossible, often due to distortion of the bladder base by a malignant prostate, then antegrade stenting (M264a, 7B173) by a radiologist should be considered.

kidney. In a particularly enlarged prostate, where there has been distortion of normal anatomy, it may be difficult or indeed impossible to introduce a guidewire or to see the ureteric orifice. It may be necessary to use a deflection mechanism (Albarrán lever) to assist in the placement of the guidewire.

Once you are satisfied that the guidewire is in a good position, the stent is introduced over

Bone pain

For my days vanish like smoke;
My bones burn like glowing embers,

Psalm 102

Eventually, the patient may present with bone pain or lethargy.

> Hormonal treatment is the first-line treatment of bone pain in prostatic cancer

Bone secondaries can be diagnosed by clinical suspicion backed up by plain X-ray or bone scan. Secondaries are typically osteosclerotic: i.e. the secondary appears more dense on X-ray, but a minority are osteolytic, i.e. less dense on X-ray. Paget's disease gives cause for confusion and the following features help distinguish osteolytic Paget's disease from lytic bone secondaries:

- thickening of the bone cortex
- coarsening of the trabecular pattern
- expansion of bone
- the pattern of spread – Paget's disease starting at the proximal end of bone and moving distally
- blade of grass/candle flame appearance in the medullary cavity of long bones.

Secondaries may emanate from other cancers, and the PSA level may assist in distinguishing them. If there is clinical doubt, a bone biopsy can be carried out and the biopsy stained for PSA.

Pathological fractures

Secondary disease can present as a pathological fracture. These fractures can heal surprisingly well, and can sometimes be the first presentation of CAP. The fracture may require bone chips to be packed into the cavity, as well as fixation at the direction of the orthopaedic surgeon.

Radiotherapy
Local radiotherapy

Radiotherapy can be given directly to the painful areas and metastases and, where facilities are available, this is an effective and surprisingly cheap option. This can be given as a single dose of 8 Gy or a larger dosage of, say, 20 Gy over a longer period of 2 or so weeks. Pain relief occurs in about three-quarters of patients. This local treatment is more effective if there are only one or two areas of pain.

Half-body radiotherapy

Wider fields can be used where there are a lot of painful metastatic areas over wider areas. Only 30% are likely to become pain-free but a useful partial response can be seen in 50%. Most patients will notice benefit within the first week or so. Patients may experience sickness or diarrhoea. Part of this disturbance is due to the breakdown of the malignant cells.

It is worth remembering that in patients with widespread marrow infiltration, painful areas can be due to marrow regeneration. Marrow scans can be used to identify patients where this is the case. It is not prudent to irradiate these areas, since they may be the only sites of red cell production left. This group of patients have a low haemoglobin and a variable reticulocyte count.

Strontium 89

Patients with hormone refractory prostate cancer often suffer considerable pain, caused by bony metastases.

Although local radiotherapy to painful areas can be employed, this is particularly difficult where secondaries are widespread.

Strontium 89 was first used as early as 1941, but has only recently become more widely used: it is a β-emitting isotope, with a half-life of 51 days. Strontium is mistaken by the body for calcium and appears to lodge preferentially at sites of increased mineral turnover. Although it is washed out of healthy bone, it is retained adjacent to osteoblastic metastases.

Clinical trials have shown that it is effective in decreasing pain, decreasing the need for pain medication and improving activity level and sleep patterns. It also improves the patient's appetite. A small percentage of patients become pain-free.

Patients who have been given strontium 89 in a UK study required less local radiotherapy or hemibody radiotherapy after strontium administration. Reduction of white cell and platelet counts were not clinically significant.

A phase III trans-Canada trial showed strontium 89 to be an important adjuvant therapy to local field radiotherapy. Of 124 patients, there was a statistically significant difference in favour of strontium, demonstrating that progression of pain was less marked in the strontium-treated arm. This was defined as the number of new sites requiring radiotherapy.[153,154]

Strontium 89 is available as a sterile aqueous solution for intravenous (IV) administration in a single outpatient injection. Each vial contains a single dose of strontium 89 chloride, of 148 MBq (4.0 mCi) in 4 ml of solution.

Pain relief usually begins between 10 and 20 days after injection and may be maintained for between 4 and 15 months (mean of 6 months).

Strontium 89 injections can be repeated on a 6-monthly basis. If the patient does not respond to the first injection however, it is unlikely that subsequent injections will work.[153–155]

Approximately 90% of strontium 89 is excreted in the urine, with the remainder being excreted through the bile.

Care should be taken in any patient with renal insufficiency.

Hormone-resistant prostate cancer

After approximately 2 years of hormone treatment, many patients will gradually develop hormone resistance in their prostate cancer. The mechanism for this is unclear, but there have been various suggestions. The most common suggestion has been that a resistant clone of cells develops and the mechanism may be due to changes in the androgen receptor or perhaps due to de-differentiation of the cells. Often, the patient feels quite well, despite a rising PSA. At this stage, it can be helpful to withdraw the hormonal treatment, to see if there is any initial response. Occasionally, withdrawal of the hormonal treatment leads to a further response, which is poorly understood, but has been identified with all of the hormonal treatments.

Hormone withdrawal

It is curious that in some patients, merely stopping their hormonal treatment causes the PSA levels to plateau. This was first observed with flutamide, but has been seen with all of the hormonal preparations.[155,156] It can be difficult to get this concept across to a patient, who is naturally worried about his gradual decline.

Systemic treatments have not been very effective at this stage.

Tannock et al[157] from Toronto achieved benefit in quality of life using mitoxantrone in these patients, but the use of steroid preparations is the main stay of treatment of this group.

Prednisolone is given in a dosage of 5 mg twice a day, either indefinitely or during a 6-month treatment period overlapping with the mitoxantrone.

At this dosage of steroid, the adrenals are suppressed (with doses over 5 mg/day), and steroid withdrawal should be gradual to avoid any complications. Patients should be issued with a card or bracelet documenting their steroid therapy.

The assistance of palliative care from physicians is to be encouraged.

Second line agents

Following this, many clinicians would change the patient to a different hormone treatment, and many have been tried. There is no single hormonal treatment which is consistently effective in this group of patients.

Some startlingly good results have been reported with estramustine phosphate. This is a combination of an oestrogen and chlormethine (mustine). The mechanism may be merely due to the high dose of oestrogen reducing testosterone, although the mustine component might produce some antimitotic changes also. It probably needs to be fully activated by hepatic metabolism. Ketoconazole, an antifungal agent, has received attention for these patients, but is not licensed in the UK.

Many of these patients are elderly, and this may be the reason why most chemotherapy agents have not proved effective. Combination chemotherapy has also been tried and to date there have been no particularly exciting regimens.

The possible palliative effects of these drugs must be balanced against the toxicity, and many patients would accept that steroid preparations remain the best symptomatic treatment.[155]

COMPLICATIONS AND THEIR TREATMENTS IN CAP

Urinary retention in prostate cancer

Some patients with prostate cancer present initially with acute retention. When a diagnosis is made, the patient is merely placed on hormonal treatment. There will be some debate as to whether it is better to perform a TURP at a relatively early stage, or to allow the patient to go home on hormonal treatment and then try a trial removal of catheter in 2–3 months. Fitness of the patient is an important guide as to which course to follow.

Channel TURP (OPCS code M6530, M651B, 7B390)
Patients may require further TURPs despite hormonal treatment. It is of interest that patients may have quite marked local disease in the prostate, or indeed just enlargement of the prostate, with a combination of BPH, and may need one or several further TURPs to allow them to pass urine. Curiously, the number of repeat TURPs does not seem to equate with survival, assuming that patients have had hormonal treatment.

It should be remembered that although the patient may have a cancer of the prostate, it may be that the symptoms are in fact due to BPH, and this will respond to a TURP.

There is no evidence that carrying out a TURP leads to dissemination of the cancer, although it is known that blood transfusion at the time of operation leads to a worse prognosis.

It is now recommended that patients receive prophylactic antibiotics prior to surgery.

Ureteric obstruction
The ureters can become obstructed and the patient presents with anuria or in renal failure.

In these patients, a nephrostomy is the first aid measure to be taken and this normally allows patients to regain some degree of well-being. At this stage, stenting of the ureters must be considered. If given the choice, most patients do elect to have the ureter or ureters stented, despite the fact that the future for them is bleak. Because the prostate has normally regrown, stenting is difficult, carried out from below and is certainly extremely difficult under local anaesthetic. Antegrade stenting may therefore be required under sedation and with the help of an interventional radiologist.

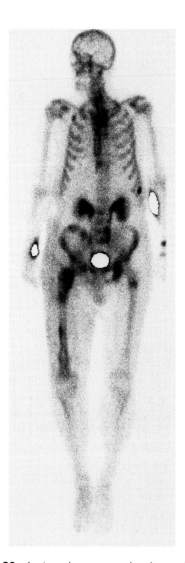

Figure 3.20 Isotope bone scan showing early skeletal metastases from primary prostate cancer. Note the bilateral hydronephrosis from ureteric obstruction.

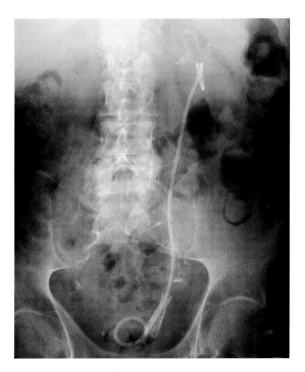

Figure 3.21 A Wallstent was inserted in the blocked left ureter. (The right ureter was also blocked by tumours). This subsequently became blocked by further tumour extension but an antegrade stent was inserted with success.

Pathological fractures

Pathological fractures often occur in patients with prostate cancer and it is surprising that they respond well to standard orthopaedic treatments. Local radiotherapy may be given and hormones can be employed if they have not already been instituted. It is gratifying that these fractures often heal up well, allowing patients to return to their former mobility.

Occasionally, large lymph nodes may be present in the pelvis and, if they are obstructing the lymphatic drainage, venous thrombosis and lymphoedema can occur. This condition can be treated by radiotherapy and, occasionally, some benefit is seen.

The presence of palpable lymphadenopathy usually implies a worse than usual prognosis.

Occasionally, patients may present with lymphadenopathy and the lymph node microscopic sections are stained with a PSA marker. A positive stain indicates the prostatic origin of the metastasis. In these patients, the use of hormonal treatment is of course the appropriate first-line therapy to be followed.

Spinal cord compression from prostate cancer

Spinal cord compression from prostate cancer is a catastrophic event for the patient, who may be condemned to a remaining lifetime of paralysis.

The patients with changing back symptoms with prostate cancer should be seen urgently and evaluated with a plain X-ray and an MR scan.

It is important that every unit has links with a neurosurgeon to discuss policy about management of these patients. It is usually the thoracic spine which is involved. Some patients also develop extradural tumour deposits.

Acute cord compression is a neurosurgical emergency caused by collapse of the vertebral body and not only angulates on to the cord but also interferes with the blood supply of the cord. It must be carefully evaluated by a neurosurgeon to see whether immediate cord decompression is appropriate. Symptoms are usually that of localised pain, with associated weakness and sensory loss and, occasionally, autonomic dysfunction.

Dexamethasone, in a dose of 4 mg four times a day, should be given immediately, unless there are very pressing contraindications, such as severe coincident infection.

This may be continued until clinical response is evident or is clearly not evident. It is usually continued during radiotherapy, and the dose must be slowly reduced due to adrenal suppression.

If the neurosurgeon feels that decompression is not indicated, the opinion of a radiotherapist should be sought.

Spinal metastases
Mechanical back pain tends to be provoked by exercise and relieved by rest.

Sudden onsets of bone pain

Bone pain in patients with malignant disease is often related to a fracture on one of the vertebrae. The other cause of pain, which is more of a serious nature, is related to pressure developing by the tumour usually compressing nervous tissue: it may or may not have root pain.

The main site of secondaries in the spine is the anterior vertebral body. The anterior motor tracts lie just behind the vertebral body and, therefore, motor loss is often the first symptom prior to sensory loss.

Because of the position of the sensory tracts lying further back, the segments may not correspond to the level of cord involvement. Occasionally, there may be a loss of sphincter control.

It is generally believed that the rate of onset of weakness and neurological deficit is associated with a poor prognosis. Conversely, patients with a slowly progressive deficit have been found to have a better prognosis. In this situation, a full nervous system examination is essential. A plain X-ray is required in many cases.

Bone scans can give confusing results, but are better in lesions that are osteoblastic (sclerotic metastases). Chemotherapy may suppress osteoblastic activity and can lead to diagnostic inaccuracy.

MR scanning gives the best visualisation of secondary disease.

Harrington divided spinal metastases into five classes:

- class 1 patients have asymptomatic spinal metastases
- class 2 patients have pain or minor neurological deficit, without bone collapse or instability
- class 3 patients have major sensory or motor loss, without significant bone involvement
- class 4 patients have pain from instability, as a result of vertebral collapse, without significant neurological deficit
- class 5 patients have significant neurological deficit and vertebral collapse or instability.[158]

The first two groups, i.e. classes 1 and 2, are usually treated by hormonal therapy, in the case of prostate cancer. Class 3 patients usually respond to radiotherapy, with or without hormonal therapy.

In bony metastases from prostate cancer, the total dose of radiation is between 40 and 50 Gy.

Surgery

Decompression is usually performed using a posterior approach. The approach, however, is determined by the pattern of bone loss and is of course the province of the neurosurgeon.

CAUSES OF DEATH IN ELDERLY PROSTATE CANCER PATIENTS

Newschaffer and his colleagues looked at the question of attribution – in other words, the cause of death – cited for patients with prostate cancer. These workers concluded that initial treatment may influence the underlying cause of death reported in vital statistics for prostate cancer patients. They found that in patients treated aggressively, the adjusted odds of other cancer causes of death were 51% higher than that in the non prostate cancer patients. This reduced to 34% in those treated with watchful waiting.[159]

COMMUNICATION WITH PATIENTS WITH CAP

Patients with CAP may well be particularly well informed about their disease. They may appear with sheaves of paper garnered from the Internet. This should be viewed by the clinician as a challenge and not as a threat to his authority. Do not presume to know everything that your patient wishes to know – you have not been in his situation! Sandblom[160] quotes the writer Anatole Broyard[161] when he was diagnosed with prostate cancer:

Like anyone who has had an extraordinary experience, I want to describe it. This seems to be a natural reflex, especially for a writer. I wanted . . . to tell people what a serious illness is like, the unprecedented ideas and fantasies it puts into your head, the unexpected qualms and quirks it introduces into your body. For a sick person, opening up your consciousness to others is like the bleeding doctors used to recommend to reduce pressure.

Once again, it has been found that we as doctors cannot fully anticipate the information needed by our patients, We must ask them.[162] Survivors' perspectives are not always those voiced in clinic.[163] Not all our patients understand what we tell them or indeed believe what we say. The use of audio and video tapes is beneficial[164] and a trained oncology nurse is invaluable.[165]

PROGNOSTIC FACTORS

The prognostic factors of prostate cancer are:

- stage
- grade
- PSA
- prostate-specific membrane antigen (PSMA)
- epithelial cadherins
- DNA content (ploidy)
- nuclear morphometry
- 12-lipoxygenase
- p53 tumour-suppressor gene
- tumour proliferative activity
- apoptosis
- neuroendocrine differentiation
- microvessel density.

CASE HISTORY (patient permission obtained)

A 67-year-old retired doctor was originally seen 9 years ago, with a history of nocturia and some morning urgency. In the past he had had a seminoma removed, followed by radiotherapy some 34 years earlier. His only other history was of prostatitis. His PSA was 10.6. He initially had a cystoscopy, which showed some mild trabeculation.

He was one of the first patients in our unit to have a transrectal ultrasound and biopsy. His biopsies proved negative and his PSA fluctuated at around 5.

He had a right inguinal hernia repaired but remained well.

Subsequent biopsies were carried out and this showed well-differentiated T1c adenocarcinoma, Gleason grades $1 + 2 = 3$. He had a negative bone scan and CT scan and a negative MR scan.

Treatment was discussed with him and the possibility of radical prostatectomy or radiotherapy was discussed. At my prompting, he was referred for a second opinion and the patient decided on a policy of watchful waiting.

He developed mild angina and had coronary angiography. He was found to have a mild proximal stenosis to the left anterior descending coronary artery, but it was felt that this was not severe and did not preclude any surgery. His PSA had risen to 13.5

He developed a change in bowel habit, and a barium enema was carried out; this was normal.

His PSA rose to 19.3 and then dropped back to 16.8. At that stage, a small 4 mm nodule became palpable and it was felt that, in view of his PSA changes, some more active treatment should be advocated.

He then sought the opinion of a radiotherapist; his PSA had further risen but was remaining stable at 22, but an MR scan showed an area of 1.8 cm × 2 cm in diameter on the left lobe of the prostate. There was no evidence of extracapsular extension or pelvic lymphadenopathy.

After further discussion, he was referred for brachytherapy. An ultrasound at that stage confirmed the tumour confined within the capsule of the prostate, with a volume of 49 ml.

He made a good recovery following his radioactive iodine seed implants, but did develop urgency, dysuria and frequency, with some rectal mucous discharge.

He then had a holiday in the Caribbean and contracted diarrhoea. This gradually settled, but he required Probanthine to control his rectal symptoms.

On his return, he was found not to be emptying his bladder and had a residual volume of around 200 ml on two occasions. It was felt that a temporary period of catheterisation would be helpful. He tolerated this for about 2 weeks.

Subsequently, he had marked urgency of defecation, which was attributed to a *Campylobacter* infection. This finally responded to erythromycin. At that stage his PSA was 1.8.

His diarrhoea persisted and sigmoidoscopy was carried out; his mucosa showed features of radiation proctitis. His PSA continued to fall to 1.3. His bowel problems gradually settled.

He is left with some residual urgency of defecation on occasions and his PSA currently is 0.89.

Practice points

The presence of prostatitis does not rule out the diagnosis of CAP.

The side effects of radiotherapy or brachytherapy are cumulative, and prior radiotherapy added to his risk of radiation proctitis.

Key points

Rectal examination remains part of physical examination – if you do not put your finger in, you will put your foot in it!

REFERENCES

1. Langstaff G. Cases of fungus haematodes, with observations. Med Chir Trans 1817; 8:272–305
2. Huggins C, Hodges CV. Studies on prostate cancer: the effect of castration, of estrogen and of androgen injection on serum phosphatases in metastatic carcinoma of the prostate. Cancer Res 1941; 1:293–297
3. Andersson L. 2000 International School of Urology and Nephrology, 9th Course, Erice, Italy. Ettore Maijorana Foundation and Centre for Scientific Culture
4. Gann PH. Interpreting recent trends in prostate cancer: incidence and mortality. Epidemiology 1997; 8:117–120
5. ONS 1998. Deaths registered in 1997 by cause. Monitor DH298/1. London: ONS, 1998
6. Annual Statistics for Scotland. Annual Recurrence. Vol. 1997. Edinburgh: Scottish Register Office, 1998
7. Gould A, Muir CS, Sharp L. Prognosis and survival in prostate cancer. In: Epidemiology of prostate disease, Garraway M (ed.). Berlin: Springer-Verlag, 1995
8. Pienta KJ. Epidemiology and etiology of prostate cancer. In: Principles and practice of genitourinary oncology, Raghavan DK, Scher HI, Leibel SA, Lange P (eds). Philadelphia: Lippincott, 1997
9. Parkin DM, Whelan SL, Ferlay J, Raymond L, Young J (eds). Cancer incidence in five continents, Vol. VII. IARC Scientific Publications No. 143. Lyons: International Agency for Research on Cancer, 1997
10. Carter HB, Piantodosi S, Isaacs JT. Clinical evidence for and implications of the multistep development of prostate cancer. J Urol 1990; 143:742–746
11. Franks LM, Durh MB. Latency and progression in tumours: the natural history of prostate cancer. Lancet 1956; 17:1037
12. Thompson I, Coltman C, Crowley J. Chemoprevention of prostate cancer: the Prostate Cancer Prevention Trial. Prostate 1997; 33:217–221
13. Ekman P. Genetic and environmental factors in prostate cancer genesis: identifying high-risk cohorts. Eur Urol 1999; 35:362–369
14. Key T. Risk factors for prostate cancer. Cancer Surv 1995; 23:63
15. Gronberg H, Damber L, Damber JE. Total food consumption and body mass index in relation to prostate cancer risk: a case-control study in Sweden with prospectively collected exposure data. J Urol 1996; 155:969–974
16. Hill P, Wynder EL, Garbaczewski L, Garnes H, Walker ARP. Diet and urinary steroids in black and white North American men and black South African men. Cancer Res 1979; 39:5101
17. Kolonel LN, Hankin JH, Yoshawa CN. Vitamin A and prostate cancer in elderly men: enhancement of risk. Cancer Res 1987; 47:2982–2985
18. Krain LS. Some epidemiologic variables in prostatic carcinoma in California. Prev Med 1974; 3:154–159
19. Rooney C, Beral V, Maconochie N, Fraser P, Davies G. Case-control study of prostatic cancer in employees of the United Kingdom Atomic Energy Authority. Br Med J 1993; 307:1391–1397
20. Eckman P, Gronberg H, Matsuyama H, Kivineva M, Bergerheim USR, Li C. Links

between genetic and environmental factors and prostate cancer risk. Prostate 1999; 39:262–268

21. Limonta P, Moretti RM, Marelli MM, Dondi D, Parenti M, Motta M. The luteinising-hormone releasing hormone receptor in human prostate cancer cells: messenger ribonucleic acid expression, molecular size, and signal transduction pathway. Endrocrinology 1999; 140(11): 5250–5256

22. Carstairs V, Morris R. Deprivation and health in Scotland. Aberdeen: Aberdeen University Press, 1991

23. Haites N, Schofield A. Inherited predisposition to uro-genital cancers. UroOncology 2001; 1(3):195–201

24. Carter BS, Beaty TH, Steinberg GD, Childs B, Walsh PC. Mendelian inheritance of familial prostate cancer. Proc Natl Acad Sci USA 1992; 89:3367–3371

25. Fox SB, Presad RA, Coleman N, et al. Prognostic value of c-erbB-2 and epidermal growth factor receptor in stage A1 (T1a) prostatic adenocarcinoma. Br J Urol 1994; 74:214–220

26. Phillips SM, Barton CM, Lee SJ, et al. Loss of the retinoblastoma susceptibility gene (RB1) is a frequent event in prostatic tumorigenesis. Br J Cancer 1994; 70:1252–1257

27. Coley CM, Barry MJ, Fleming C, Wasson JH, Fahs MC, Oesterling JE. Should Medicare provide reimbursement for prostate-specific antigen testing for early detection of prostate cancer? Part II: early detection strategies. Urology 1995; 46:125–141

28. Epstein JI, Walsh PC, Carmichael M, Brendler CB. Pathologic and clinical findings to predict tumour extent of non palpable (stage T1c) prostate cancer. JAMA 1994; 271:368–374

29. Richie JP, Catalona WJ, Ahmann FR, et al. Effect of patient age on early detection of prostate cancer with serum prostate-specific antigen and digital rectal examination. Urology 1993; 42:365–374

30. Chodak GW, Keller P, Schoenberg HW. Assessment of screening for prostate cancer, using the digital rectal examination. J Urol 1989; 141:1136–1138

31. Wang ML, Valenzuela L, Murphy GP, Chu T. Purification of human prostate specific antigen. Invest Urol 1979; 17:159–163

32. Stamey TA, Yang N, Hay AR. Prostate specific antigen as a serum marker for adenocarcinoma of the prostate. N Engl J Med 1987; 317:909–916

33. Lilja U. Structure and function of prostatic and seminal vesicle-secreted proteins involved in the gelation and liquefaction of human semen. Scand J Lab Invest 1988; 48(suppl):13–17

34. Catalona WJ, Smith DS, Ratliff TL, Basler JW. Detection of organ confined prostate cancer is increased through prostate specific antigen based screening. JAMA 1993; 270:948–954

35. Oesterling JE, Jacobsen SJ, Chute CG, et al. Serum prostate specific antigen in a community-based population of healthy men. Establishment of age specific rates. JAMA 1993; 270(7):860–864

36. Bangma CH, Kranse R, Blijenburg BG, Schroder FH. The value of screening tests in the detection of prostate cancer. Part II. Retrospective analysis of free/total prostate-specific analysis ratio, age specific reference ranges and PSA density. Urology 1995; 46(6):779–784

37. Lilja H, Cockett AT, Abrahamsson PA. Prostate specific antigen predominantly forms a complex with alpha 1-antichymotrypsin in blood. Implications for procedures to measure prostate specific antigen in serum. Cancer 1992; 70(1 suppl):230–234

38. Bangma CH, Rietbergen JB, Kranse R, Blijenburg BG, Pettersson K, Schroder FH. The free-to-total prostate specific antigen ratio improves the specificity of prostate specific antigen in screening for prostate cancer in the general population. J Urol 1997; 157(6): 2191–2196

39. Catalona WJ, Smith DS, Ratliff TL, et al. Measurement of prostate-specific antigen in serum as a screening test for prostate cancer. N Engl J Med 1991; 324:1156–1161

40. Brawer MK, Chetner MP, Beatie J, Buchner DM, Vessella RL, Lange PH. Screening for prostatic carcinoma with prostate specific antigen. J Urol 1992; 1473(3:2):841–845

41. Richie JP, Catalona WJ, Ahmann FR, et al. Effect of patient age on early detection of prostate cancer with serum prostate-antigen and digital rectal examination. Urology 1993; 42:365–374

42. Catalona WJ, Richie JP, Ahmann FR, et al. Comparison of digital rectal examination and serum prostate specific antigen in the early detection of prostate cancer: results of a multicentre clinical trial of 6,630 men. J Urol 1994; 151:1283–1290

43. Mettlin C, Murphy GP, Ray P, et al. American Cancer Society–National Prostate Cancer Detection Project. Results from multiple examinations using transrectal ultrasound, digital

rectal examination and prostate specific antigen. Cancer 1993; 71(3 suppl):891–898

44. Catalona WJ, Smith DS, Ratliff TL, Basler JW. Detection of organ-confined prostate cancer is increased through prostatic-specific antigen-based screening. JAMA 1993; 270:948–954

45. Aus G, Ahlgren G, Bergdahl S, Hugosson J. Infection after transrectal core biopsies of the prostate – risk factors and antibiotic prophylaxis. Br J Urol 1996; 77:851–855

46. Collins GN, Lloyd SN, Hehir M, McKelvie GB. Multiple transrectal ultrasound-guided biopsies – true morbidity and patient acceptance. Br J Urol 1997; 79:460–463

47. Hodge KK, McNeal JE, Terris MK, Stamey TA. Random systematic versus directed ultrasound guided transrectal core biopsies of the prostate. J Urol 1989; 142:71–75

48. Stamey TA. Making the most out of six systemic sextant biopsies. Urology 1995; 45: 541–544

49. Schroder FH, Hermanek P, Denis L, Fair WR, Gospodarowicz MK, Pavone-Macaluso M. The TNM classification of prostate cancer. Prostate 1992; 4:129–138

50. Hermanek P, Hutter RVP, Sobin LH, Wagner G, Wittekind CH. TNM atlas, 4th edn, UICC. Berlin: Springer, 1997

51. Aus G, Abbou CC, Pacik D, et al. Guidelines on prostate cancer. Brussels: European Association of Urology, 2000

52. Bostwick DG. Staging prostate cancer – 1997; current methods & limitations. Eur Urol 1997; 32:(suppl 3):2–14

53. Cooner W, Mosley R, Rutherford CJ, et al. Prostate cancer detection in a clinical urological practice by ultrasonography, digital rectal examination and prostate-specific antigen. J Urol 1990; 143:1146–1152

54. Lee F, Littrup PJ, Torp-Pederson ST, et al. Prostate cancer: comparison of transrectal US and DRE for screening. Radiology 1988; 168:389–394

55. Catalona W, Smith D, Ratcliff T, et al. Measurement of prostate–specific antigen in serum as a screening test for prostate cancer. N Engl J Med 1991; 324:1156–1161

56. Catalona WJ, Richie JP, Ahmann FR, et al. Comparison of digital rectal examination and serum prostate-specific antigen in the early detection of prostate cancer: results of a multicentre clinical trial of 6,630 men. J Urol 1994; 151:1283–1290

57. Mettlin C, Lee F, Drago J, et al. The American Cancer Society National Prostate Cancer Detection Project: findings on the detection of early prostate cancer in 2425 men. Cancer 1991; 67:2949–2958

58. Fenely MR. Does screening for prostate cancer identify clinically important disease? Ann R Coll Surg Engl 1999; 81:207–214

59. Wasson JH, Cushman CC, Bruskewitz RC, Littenberg B, Mulley AG Jr, Wennberg JE. A structured literature review for localized prostate cancer. Arch Fam Med 1993; 2:487–493

60. Coley CC, Barry MJ, Fleming C, Fahs MC, Mulley AG. Ann Int Med 1997; 126:468–479

61. Essink-Bot ML, Koning Hjde, Nijs HGT, Kirkels WJ, Maas PJ van der, Schroder FH. Short-term effects of population-based screening for prostate cancer on health-related quality of life. J Natl Cancer Inst 1998; 90(12):925–931

62. Labrie F, Candas B, Dupont A, et al. Screening decreases prostate cancer death: first analysis of the 1988 Quebec prospective randomized controlled trial. Prostate 1999; 38:83–91

63. Boer R. Quebec randomized controlled trial on prostate cancer screening shows no evidence for mortality reduction [Letter to the editor]. Prostate 1999; 40:130–131.

64. Alexander FE, Prescott RJ. Reply to Labrie, et al. Results of the mortality of the Quebec Randomized/controlled trial (RCT). Prostate 1999; 40:135–137

65. Labrie F, Candas B, Dupont A, et al. Screening decreases prostate cancer death: first analysis of the 1988 Quebec prospective randomized controlled trial. Prostate 1999; 38:83–91.

66. Beemsterboer PMM, Kranse R, Koning HJ de, Habbema JDF, Schroder FH. Changing role for 3 screening modalities in the European Randomised Study of Screening for Prostate Cancer (Rotterdam). Int J Cancer 1998; 84(4):437–441

67. Horninger W, Reissigl A, Rogatsch H, et al. Prostate cancer screening in the Tyrol, Austria: experience and results. Eur J Cancer 2000; 36(10):1322–1335

68. McNeal JE. The zonal anatomy of the prostate. Prostate 1981; 2(1):35–49

69. McNeal JE. Normal histology of the prostate. Am J Surg Pathol 1988; 12:619–633

70. Mostoffi FK, Price EB. Tumors of the male genital system. Washington. AFIP, 1973

71. Ittman M, Wieczorek R, Heller P, et al. Alterations of the p53 and MDM-2 genes are

infrequent in clinically localized, stage B prostate adenocarcinomas. Am J Pathol 1994; 145:287–293

72. Hamdy FC, Johnson MI, Robson CN. Prostate cancer. In: The scientific basis of urology, Mundy AR, Fitzpatrick JM, Neal DE, George NJ (eds). Oxford: Isis Medical Media, 1999

73. Gnanapragasam VJ, Robson CN, Leung HY, Neal DE. Androgen receptor signalling in the prostate. BJU Int 2000; 86:1001–1013

74. McNeal JE. Origin and development of carcinoma in the prostate. Cancer 1969; 23:24–33

75. Bostwick DG. Prostatic intraepithelial neoplasia (PIN). Urology 1989; 34(suppl):16–22

76. Brawer MK, Bigler SA, Sohlberg OE, Nagle RB, Lange PH. Significance of prostatic intraepithelial neoplasia on prostate needle biopsy. Urology 1991; 38:103–107

77. Gleason DF. Histologic grading of prostate cancer: a perspective. Hum Pathol 1992; 23:273–279

78. Albertsen PC, Fryback DG, Storer BE, Kolon TF, Fine J. Long-term survival among men with conservatively treated localized prostate cancer. JAMA 1995; 274:626–631

79. George NJR. Natural history of localised prostatic cancer managed by conservative therapy alone. Lancet 1988; 1:494–497

80. Johansson JE Andersson SO, Krusemo UB. Natural history of localised prostatic cancer. Lancet 1989; I:799–803

81. Johansson JE. Watchful waiting for early stage prostate cancer. Urology 1994; 43:138–142

82. Johansson JE, Adami HO, Andersson SO, Bergstrom R, Holmberg L, Krusemo UB. High 10-year survival rate in patients with early, untreated prostatic cancer. JAMA 1992; 267:2191–2196

83. Adolffson J, Steineck G, Whitmore WF Jr. Recent results of management of palpable clinically localized prostate cancer. Cancer 1993; 72:43–55

84. Jones GW. Prospective conservative management of localized prostate cancer. Cancer 1992; 70(suppl):307–310

85. Aus G. Prostate cancer: mortality and morbidity after non-curative treatment with aspects on diagnosis and treatment. Scand J Urol Nephrol 1994; 167(suppl):1–41

86. Carter HB, Pearson JD, Metter EJ, et al. Longitudinal evaluation of prostate-specific antigen levels in men with and without prostate disease. JAMA 1992; 267:2215–2220

87. Gann PH, Hennekens CH, Stampfer MJ. A prospective evaluation of plasma prostate-specific antigen for detection of prostate cancer. JAMA 1995; 273:289–294

88. Albertsen PC, Fryback DG, Storer BE, et al. Long-term survival among men with conservatively treated localized prostate cancer. JAMA 1995; 274:626

89. Chodak GW, Thirsted RA, Gerber GS, et al. Results of conservative management of clinically localized prostate cancer. N Engl J Med 1994; 330:242–248

90. Rinker-Schaeffer CW, Welch DR, Sokoloff M. Defining the biologic role of genes that regulate prostate cancer metastasis. Curr Opin Urol 2000; 10:397–401

91. Eichel L, Messing E. The timing of hormonal treatment for prostate cancer. Curr Opin Urol 2000; 10:403–407

92. Lu-Yao G, Yao SL. Population-based study of long-term survival in patients with clinically localised prostate cancer. Lancet 1997; 349(9056):906–910

93. Walsh PC, Lepor H, Eggleston JC. Radical prostatectomy with preservation of sexual function: anatomical and pathological considerations. Prostate 1983; 4:473–485

94. Middleton RG, Thompson IM, Austenfield MS, et al. Prostate cancer clinical guidelines panel summary report on the management of clinically localized prostate cancer. J Urol 1995; 154:2144–2148

95. Talcott JA, Rieker P, Propert KJ, et al. Long-term complications of treatment for early prostate cancer: two-year follow up in a prospective multi-institutional outcomes study (abstract). J Clin Oncol 1996; 15:252

96. D'Amico AV, Whittington R, Malkowicz B, et al. Biochemical outcome after radical prostatectomy, external beam radiation therapy, or interstitial radiation therapy for clinically localized prostate cancer. JAMA 1998; 280:969–974

97. Partin AW, Kattan MW, Subong EN, et al. Combination of prostate-specific antigen, clinical stage, and Gleason score to predict pathological stage of localized prostate cancer. A multi-institutional update. JAMA 1997; 277:1445–1457

98. Albertsen PC, Hanley JA, Gleason DF, Barry MJ. Competing risk analysis of men aged 55 to 74 years at diagnosis managed conservatively for clinically localized prostate cancer. JAMA 1998; 280(11):975–980

99. Trapasso JG, DeKernion JB, Smith RB, Dorey F.

Incidence and significance of detectable levels of serum prostate specific antigen after radical prostatectomy. J Urol 1994; 152:1821–1825

100. Walsh PC, Partin AW, Epstein JI. Cancer control & quality of life following anatomical radical retropubic prostatectomy: results at 10 years. J Urol 1994; 152:1831–1836

101. Walsh PC. Anatomic radical retropubic prostatectomy. In: Campbells urology, 7th edn, Walsh et al (eds). Philadelphia: WB Saunders, 1997

102. Walsh PC. Anatomic radical prostatectomy: evolution of the surgical technique. J Urol 1998; 160:2418–2424

103. Harnden P, Parkinson MC. Macroscopic examination of prostatic specimens. J Clin Pathol 1995; 48:693–700

104. Feldman HA, Goldstein I, Hatzichristou DG, et al. Impotence and its medical and psychological correlates: results of the Massachusetts Male Aging Study. J Urol 1994; 15:54–61

105. Thuroff JW. Editor of laparoscopic radical prostatectomy: feasibility studies or the future standard technique? Curr Opin Urol 2000; 10(5):363–364

106. Rassweiler J, Sentker L, Seeman O, et al. Laparoscopic radical prostatectomy: technique and early experience [In German]. Akt Urol 2000; 31:237–245

107. Guillonneau B, Chathelineau X, Barret E, et al. Morbidity of laparoscopic radical prostatectomy; evaluation after 210 procedures [abstract]. J Urol 2000; 163(suppl):140

108. Babaian RJ, Kojima M, Saitoh M, Ayala A. Detection of residual prostate cancer after external radiotherapy. Cancer 1995; 75:2158–2160

109. Crook J, Robertson S, Collin G, Zaleski V, Esche B. Clinical relevance of trans-rectal ultrasound, biopsy, and serum prostate specific antigen following external beam radiotherapy for carcinoma of the prostate. Int J Radiat Oncol Biol Phys 1993; 26:31–37

110. Crook J, Malone S, Perry G, Bahadur Y, Robertson S, Abdolell M. Postradiotherapy prostate biopsies: what do they really mean? Int J Radiat Oncol Biol Phys 2000; 48(2):355–367

111. Crook J. Biopsy outcome after definitive radiotherapy. In: Radiotherapy of prostate cancer, Greco C, Zelefsky MJ (eds). Amsterdam: Harwood Academic Publishers, 2000

112. Crook JM, Bahadur YA, Robertson SJ, Perry GA, Esche BA. Evaluation of radiation effect, tumour differentiation and prostate specific antigen staining in sequential prostate biopsies after external beam radiotherapy for patients with prostate carcinoma. Cancer 1997; 79:81–89

113. Crook JM, Bahadur YA, Perry GA, Malone SC, Robertson SJ. Radiotherapy for prostate cancer: results of systematic biopsies for 479 patients. J Urol 1998; 159:A239

114. Prestidge BR, Kaplan I, Cox RS, Bagshaw MA. Predictors of survival after a positive post-irradiation prostate biopsy. Int J Radiat Oncol Biol Phys 1994; 28:17–22

115. Perez CS, Michalski J, Brown KC, Lockett MA. Non randomized evaluation of pelvic lymph node radiation in localized carcinoma of the prostate. Int J Radiat Oncol Biol Phys 1996; 36:573–584

116. Bolla M, Gonzalez D, Warde P, et al. Immediate hormonal therapy improves locoregional control and survival in patients with locally advanced prostate cancer. Results of a randomised phase III clinical trial of the EORTC Radiotherapy and Genitourinary Tract Cancer Cooperative Groups. Proc Am Soc Clin Oncol 1996; 15(abstract):591

117. Pilepich MV, Caplan R, Al-Sarraf M, et al. Phase III trial of hormonal cytoreduction in conjunction with definitive radiotherapy in locally advanced prostate carcinoma – the emerging role in PSA in the assessment of outcome. Int J Radiat Oncol Biol Phys 1993; 27(suppl 1):246

118. Holm HH. History of interstitial brachytherapy of prostatic cancer. Sem Surg Oncol 1997; 13:431–437

119. Ash D, Bottomley DM, Carey BM. Prostate brachytherapy. Prostate Cancer and Prostatic Diseases 1998; 1:185–188

120. Beyer DC, Priestley JB. Biochemical disease-free survival following iodine 125 prostate implantation. Int J Radiat Oncol Biol Phys 1997; 37:559–563

121. Prestidge BR, Hoak DC, Grimm PD, Ragde H, Cavanagh W, Blasko JC. Posttreatment biopsy results following interstitial brachytherapy in early-stage prostate cancer. Int J Radiat Oncol Biol Phys 1997; 37:31–39

122. Ragde H, Blasko JC, Grimm PD, et al. Brachytherapy for clinically localized prostate cancer: results at 7–8 year follow-up. Sem Surg Oncol 1997; 13:438–443

123. Lee F, Bahn DK, Badalament RA, et al. Cryosurgery for prostate cancer: improved glandular ablation by use of 6 to 8 cryoprobes. Urology 1999; 54(10):135–140

124. Larson TR, Robertson DW, Corica A, Bostwick

DG. In vivo interstitial temperature mapping of the human prostate during cryosurgery with correlation to histopathologic outcomes. Urology 2000; 55(40):547–552

125. Schulman CC, Altwein JE, Zlotta AR. Treatment options after failure of local curative treatments in prostate cancer: a controversial issue. BJU Int 2000; 86:1014–1022

126. Messing EM, Manola J, Sarosdy M, et al. Immediate hormonal therapy compared with observation after radical prostatectomy and pelvic lymphadenopathy in men with node-positive prostate cancer. N Engl J Med 1999; 341:1781–1788

127. Zagars GK, Von Eschenbach AC. Prostate-specific antigen: an important marker for prostate cancer treated by external beam radiation therapy. Cancer 1993; 72:538–548

128. Crook JM, Choan E, Perry GA, Robertson S, Esche BA. Serum prostate-specific antigen profile following radiotherapy for prostate cancer: implications for patterns of failure and definition of cure. Urology 1998; 51:566–572

129. Lerner SE, Blute ML, Zincke H. Critical evaluation of salvage surgery for radiorecurrent/resistant prostate cancer. J Urol 1995; 154:1103–1109

130. Gleave ME, Goldenberg LS, et al. Maximal biochemical and pathological downstaging requires 8 months of neoadjuvant hormonal therapy prior to radical prostatectomy. J Urol 1995; 153:392A

131. Kirk D and The MRC Prostate Cancer Working Party and Investigators Group. Immediate versus deferred treatment study. Br J Urol 1997; 79:235–246

132. Anderson JB. Early versus deferred hormone therapy. Eur Urol 1999; 36(suppl 2):9–13

133. Schulman CC. The aging male: a challenge for urologists. Curr Opin Urol 2000; 10:337–345

134. Veterans Administration Co-operative Urological Research Group: Treatment and survival of patients with cancer of the prostate. Surg Gynecol Obstet 1967; 124:1011–1017

135. Cox RL, Crawford ED. Estrogens in the treatment of prostate cancer. J Urol 1995; 154:1991–1998

136. Huggins C, Stevens RE, Hodges CV. Studies on prostatic cancer. II. The effects of castration on advanced carcinoma of the prostate gland. Arch Surg 1941; 43:209–223

137. Huggins C, Stevens RE, Hodges CV. Studies on prostatic cancer; effects of castration on advanced carcinoma of prostate. J Urol 1941; 46:997–1006

138. Byar DP. Proceedings: Veterans Administrative Cooperative Urological Research Group's studies of cancer of the prostate. Cancer 1973; 32:1126–1130

139. McClinton S, Moffat L, Ludbrook A. The cost of bilateral orchiectomy as a treatment for prostatic carcinoma. Br J Urol 1989; 63:209–213

140. Peeling WB. Phase III studies to compare goserelin (Zoladex) with orchiectomy and with diethylstilbestrol in treatment of prostatic carcinoma. Urology 1989; 33(suppl):45–52

141. Vogelzang NJ, Chodak GW, Soloway MS, et al. Goserelin versus orchiectomy in the treatment of advanced prostate cancer: final results of a randomized trial. Zoladex Prostate Study Group. Urology 1995; 46:220–226

142. Kolvenbag GJCM, Newling D, McLeod DG, Debruyne F. UroOncology 2001; 1(2):73–90

143. Iversen P, Tyrrell CJ, Kaisary AV, et al. Bicalutamide ('Casodex') 150 mg monotherapy compared with castration in patients with non-metastatic locally advanced prostate cancer: 6.3 years' follow-up. J Urol 2000; 164:1579–1582

144. Eisenberger MA, Blumenstein BA, Crawford ED. Bilateral orchidectomy with or without flutamide for metastatic prostate cancer. N Engl J Med 1998; 339:1036–1042

145. Schroder FH, Collette L. Prostate cancer treated by anti-androgens: is sexual function preserved? Br J Cancer 2000, 82(2):283–290

146. Stone P, Hardy J, Hoddart R, Hern RA, Richards M. Fatigue in patients with prostate cancer receiving hormone therapy, Eur J Cancer 2000; 36:1134–1141

147. Anon. Maximum androgen blockade in advanced prostate cancer; an overview of 22 randomised trials with 3283 deaths in 5710 patients. Lancet 1995; 346:246–269

148. Prostate Cancer Triallists' Collaborative Group. Maximum androgen blockade in advanced prostate cancer: an overview of 22 randomised trials with 3283 deaths in 5710 patients. Lancet 1995; 346:265–269

149. Denis LJ, Keuppens F, Smith PH, et al for the EORTC Genito-Urinary Tract Cancer Cooperative Group and the EORTC Data Center: Maximal androgen blockade: final analysis of EORTC phase III trial 30853. Eur Urol 1998; 33:144–151

150. Bennett CL, Tosteson TD, Schmitt B. Maximum androgen blockade with medical or surgical

castration in advanced prostate cancer: a meta-analysis of nine published randomized controlled trials and 4128 patients using flutamide. Prost Cancer Prost Dis 1999; 2:4–8

151. Higano CS, Ellis W, Russell K, Lange PH. Intermittent androgen suppression with leuprolide and flutamide for prostate cancer: a pilot study. Urology 1996; 48:800–804

152. Bruchovsky N, Goldenberg SL, Gleave M, Rennie P, Akakura K, Sato N. Intermittent therapy for prostate cancer. Endocrine-Related Cancer 1997; 4:153–177

153. Crawford ED, Kozlowski JM, Debruyne FMJ, et al. The use of strontium 89 for pallation of pain from bone metastases, associated with hormone-refractory prostate cancer. Urology 1994; 44(4):481–485

154. Porter AT, McEwan AJB, Powe JE, et al. Results of a randomized phase-iii trial to evaluate the efficacy of strontium-89 adjuvant to local field external beam irradiation in the management of endocrine resistant metastatic prostate cancer. Int J Radiat Oncol Biol Phys 1993; 25(5):805–812

155. Kelly WK, Slovin S, Scher HI. Steroid hormone withdrawal syndromes: pathophysiology and clinical significance. Urol Clin North Am 1997; 24:421–431

156. Isaacs JT. The biology of hormone refractory prostate cancer: Why does it develop? Urol Clin North Am, Pienta KJ (ed.) 1999; 26:263–273

157. Tannock IF, Osoba D, Stockler MR, et al. Chemotherapy with mitoxantrone plus prednisone or prednisone alone for symptomatic hormone-resistant prostate cancer: a Canadian randomised trial with palliative endpoints. J Clin Oncol 1996; 14:1756–1764

158. Harrington KD. Metastatic disease of the spine. J Bone Joint Surg (Am) 1986; 68:1110

159. Newschaffer CJ, Otani K, McDonald K, Penberthy LT. Causes of death in elderly prostate cancer patients in a comparison nonprostate cancer cohort. J Natl Cancer Inst 2000; 92(8): 613–621

160. Sandblom P. Creativity and disease, 12th edn. London: Marion Boyars, 1992

161. Broyard A. NY Times Book Review, 1990

162. Feldman-Stewart D, Kocouski N, McConnell BA, et al. What questions do patients with curable prostate cancer want answered? Med Decis Making 2000; 20:7–19

163. Fitch MI. Survivors' perspectives on the impact of prostate cancer: implications of oncology nurses. Can Oncol Nurse J 1999; 9:23–24

164. Schapira MM, Meade C, Nattinger AB. Enhanced decision-making: the use of a video-tape decision-aid for patients with prostate cancer. Patient Education and Counselling 1996; 30:119–127

165. Wolf AMD, Schorling JB. Preferences of elderly men for prostate-specific antigen screening and the impact of informed consent. J Gerontol Med Sci 1998; 53A:M195–M200

FURTHER READING

Prostate cancer

Aus G, Abbou CC, Pacik D, et al. Guidelines on prostate cancer. Brussels: European Association of Urology, 2000

Coptcoat M. The management of advanced prostate cancer. London: Blackwell, 1996

Crawford ED, Eisenberger MA, McLeod DG, et al. A controlled trial of leuprolide with and without flutamide in prostatic carcinoma. N Engl J Med 1989; 321:419–424

Eastham JA, Scardino PT. Radical prostatectomy. In: Campbells urology, 7th edn, Walsh et al (eds). Philadelphia: WB Saunders, 1997

Hamdy FC, Johnson MI, Robson CN. Prostate cancer. In: The scientific basis of urology, Mundy AR, Fitzpatrick JM, Neal DE, George NJ (eds). Oxford: Isis Medical Media, 1999

Lawton CA, Won M, Pilepich MV, et al. Long-term treatment sequelae following external beam irradiation for adenocarcinoma of the prostate: analysis of RTOG studies 7506 and 7706. Int J Radiat Oncol Biol Phys 1991; 21:935–939

The Royal College of Radiologists Clinical Oncology Network. Clinical Oncology 1999; 11:s55–s8

Economics

Chamberlain J, Melia S, Moss S, Brown J. Report prepared for the health technology assessment panel of the NHS executive on the diagnosis, management, treatment and costs of prostate cancer in England and Wales. Br J Urol 1997; 79(suppl 3): 1–32

Litwin, Mark S. Cost of treating genitourinary cancer. In: Principles and practice of genitourinary oncology, Raghavan D, Scher HI, Leibel S, Lange P (eds). Philadelphia: Lippincott, 1997

McClinton S, Moffat L, Ludbrook A. The cost of bilateral orchiectomy as a treatment for prostatic carcinoma. Br J Urol 1989; 63:209–213

Otnes B, Harvei S, Fossa SD. The burden of prostate cancer from diagnosis to death. Br J Urol 1995; 76:587–594

Shiell A, Pettipher C, Raynes N, Wright K. Economic approaches to measuring quality of life. In: Quality of life, Baldwin S, Godfrey C, Propper C (eds). London: Routledge, 1992

Classic papers

Byar DP. Proceedings: Veterans Administrative Cooperative Urological Research Group's studies of cancer of the prostate. Cancer 1973; 32: 1126–1130

Catalona WJ, Smith DS, Ratliff TL, Basler JW. Detection of organ confined prostate cancer is increased through prostate specific antigen based screening. JAMA 1993; 270:948–954

Crawford ED, Eisenberger MA, McLeod DG, et al. A controlled trial of leuprolide with and without flutamide in prostatic carcinoma. N Engl J Med 1989; 321:419–424

Eisenberger MA, Blumenstein BA, Crawford ED, et al. Bilateral orchidectomy with or without flutamide for metastatic prostate cancer. N Engl J Med 1998; 339:1036–1042

Gleason DF, Veterans Cooperative Urological Research Group. Histologic grading and clinical staging of prostate carcinoma. Urologic pathology. In: The prostate, Tannenbaum M (ed.). Philadelphia: Lea & Febiger, 1977; pp. 171–197

Huggins C, Hodges CV. Studies on prostate cancer: the effect of castration, of estrogen and of androgen injection on serum phosphatases in metastatic carcinoma of the prostate. Cancer Res 1941; 1:293–297

Kirk D and The MRC Prostate Cancer Working Party and Investigators Group. Immediate versus deferred treatment study. Br J Urol 1997; 79: 235–246

McNeal JE. Origin and development of carcinoma in the prostate. Cancer 1969; 23:24–33

Stamey TA, Yang N, Hay AR, McNeal JE, Freiha FS, Redwine E. Prostate specific antigen as a serum marker for adenocarcinoma of the prostate. N Engl J Med 1987; 317:909–916

The Veterans Administration Cooperative Urological Research Group. Treatment and survival of patients with cancer of the prostate. Surg Gynaecol Obst 1967; 124:1011–1017

Walsh PC, Lepor H, Eggleston JC. Radical prostatectomy with preservation of sexual function: anatomical and pathological considerations. Prostate 1983; 4:473–485

Whitmore WF. The natural history of prostatic cancer. Cancer 1973; 32:1104–1112

4

Bladder cancer

Grubbing weeds from gravel paths with broken dinner-knives.

Rudyard Kipling 1865–1936[1]

GENERAL COMMENTARY

Bladder cancer was one of the first cancers to be recognised as an industrial cancer. The association with bladder cancer was first recorded in aniline dye workers by Rehn[2] in 1895. The environmental aspects are dealt with fully in Chapter 1.

Bladder cancer has a relatively strong association with smoking and, because more women are now smoking, the numbers of bladder cancers are increasing in women. Schistosomiasis predisposes to bladder cancer, more often to squamous carcinoma.

The vast majority of bladder cancers are cancers of the transitional cell epithelium. A further 5% are squamous cell carcinomas (ICD-10:C679e) and the remainder are a mixture of adenocarcinomas (2%; ICD-10: C679d), small cell carcinomas and undifferentiated carcinomas. There are a number of rare cancers, such as soft tissue sarcoma, carcinosarcoma, lymphomata and phaeochromocytoma.[3]

INCIDENCE

Male:female = 3:1.[3] The incidence[4] of bladder cancer is shown in Table 4.1.

MORTALITY

The relative survival rates from bladder cancer in several countries are compared in Table 4.2 and Figure 4.1.

AETIOLOGY – NON-GENETIC

Exposure to industrial carcinogens is associated with bladder cancer (see Chapter 1). A wide variety of occupations are exposed to chemicals, including:

- barbers
- chemical workers
- dental technicians
- dry cleaners
- furniture makers using solvents
- gardeners
- hairdressers
- leather workers
- painters
- petroleum workers
- plumbers
- rubber and tyre workers.[3]

Tobacco smoking predisposes to bladder cancer and also increases absorption of some carcinogens. There is a direct relationship with an increasing risk with an increased cigarette consumption.[5] Some patients have an increased activation of a hepatic acetylation mechanism. If you are a rapid acetylator, you can inactivate certain carcinogens faster and this reduces the

Table 4.1 Age-standardised incidence rates and standard errors per 100,000 for cancer of bladder (ICD-9 188)

Country	Male (SE)		Female (SE)	
Zimbabwe, Harare: African	13.2	1.88	12.5	2.17
Zimbabwe, Harare: European	27.4	5.02	7.8	2.59
Argentina, Concordia	9.1	1.81	3.9	1.07
Brazil, Goiania	18.6	1.22	2.6	0.49
Ecuador, Quito	5.1	0.57	1.5	0.27
Peru, Lima	5.5	0.38	1.7	0.20
US, Puerto Rico	8.5	0.33	2.7	0.17
Uruguay, Montevideo	19.7	0.88	3.7	0.31
Canada	18.7	0.15	5.0	0.07
US, SEER:[a] White	24.0	0.20	6.2	0.09
US, SEER: Black	11.1	0.47	4.3	0.24
China, Shanghai	6.9	0.18	1.8	0.08
Hong Kong	14.5	0.32	4.3	0.16
India, Bombay	4.8	0.22	1.2	0.11
Israel: all Jews	25.2	0.49	5.3	0.21
Israel: non-Jews	13.1	1.22	1.4	0.35
Japan, Hiroshima	12.9	0.67	2.8	0.27
Korea, Kangwa	3.1	0.99	1.3	0.63
Kuwait: non-Kuwaitis	17.5	3.29	4.2	1.25
Kuwait: Kuwaitis	7.0	1.13	2.5	0.81
Philippines, Manila	4.9	0.36	1.5	0.17
Singapore: Chinese	7.7	0.43	2.0	0.20
Vietnam: Hanoi	1.7	0.28	0.2	0.09
Austria, Tyrol	28.3	1.76	6.6	0.52
Czech Republic	15.4	0.22	3.2	0.09
Denmark	27.9	0.38	7.7	0.19
Finland	15.2	0.28	3.1	0.11
France, Calvados	23.9	1.14	3.7	0.39
Germany: Eastern States	19.2	0.32	3.4	0.11
Germany: Saarland	23.1	0.78	5.2	0.30
Ireland, Southern	12.2	0.87	4.0	0.49
Italy, Genoa	38.3	1.12	6.7	0.42
The Netherlands	15.2	0.20	3.0	0.08
Poland, Warsaw City	13.1	0.56	3.0	0.23
Spain, Zaragoza	22.4	0.84	2.7	0.26
Sweden	17.3	0.22	4.6	0.11
UK, England and Wales	20.3	0.13	5.7	0.07
UK, Scotland	22.9	0.36	7.3	0.18
Yugoslavia, Vojvodina	11.5	0.41	2.6	0.17
South Australia	20.6	0.66	5.9	0.34
US, Hawaii: White	24.2	1.66	5.9	0.83
US, Hawaii: Japanese	10.9	1.00	3.3	0.53
US, Hawaii: Hawaiian	3.9	1.00	3.2	0.86
US, Hawaii: Filipino	5.4	1.06	2.7	0.77
US, Hawaii: Chinese	9.6	1.86	2.7	0.99

[a]SEER = Surveillance, Epidemiology and End Results programme.

Table 4.2 International comparison of survival from bladder cancer (ICD-9 188). Relative survival (%) at 5 years, all ages, patients diagnosed 1985–89		
	Survival (%)	
Country	**Males**	**Females**
USA	83.9	75.7
Denmark	51.0	44.0
Finland	70.0	65.0
France	62.0	55.0
Germany	76.0	62.0
Italy	69.0	64.0
Netherlands	67.0	49.0
Spain	72.0	70.0
Sweden	75.0	70.0
England & Wales	62.0	57.0
Scotland	65.0	58.7

measured risk but most people are unaware of their acetylator status. It does not afford total protection however.[6]

Substances associated with bladder cancer

- Aluminium production products
- Auramine and magenta manufacture products
- Rubber industry products
- Leather industry products
- 4-Aminobiphenyl
- Benzidine
- Naphthylamine.

AETIOLOGY – GENETIC

Abnormalities have been reported on chromosomes 3, 5, 7, 9 and 11. Main abnormalities: 9p (source of cyclin-dependent kinase) and 11p.

Loss of heterozygosity in chromosome 17, the site of the p53 gene, is found in up to 50% of patients with carcinoma in situ (CIS)[7]

Changes in the retinoblastoma gene (*rb*) on the long arm of 13(q) are not common, but where seen, are associated with a poor prognosis.[8–10]

RISK FACTORS

- Age
- Smoking (×4 risk)
- Occupational exposure to aniline dyes and aromatic amines
- Phenacetin abuse (now much rarer than previously)
- Cyclophosphamide treatment in past.[3]

NATURAL HISTORY

Most new bladder cancers are well or moderately differentiated and are said to be superficial at presentation. The majority (50–70%) recur following endoscopic resection. When they recur, most remain well differentiated but 20% are high grade. About 10% develop invasive characteristics and may metastasise.

If untreated, the tumour becomes invasive, eroding through the lamina propria and into detrusor muscle.

The tumour spreads to regional lymph nodes in the pelvis, especially the obturator nodes and the iliac nodes. The tumour can metastasise to lungs, liver and brain.

Tumours may spread within the bladder, and this can occur after tumour resection, especially if the bladder has not been properly irrigated.

About 30% present *de novo* with muscle invasive disease and about half have occult metastases.[11]

CLINICAL PRESENTATION

- Painless haematuria – usually frank.
- Irritative symptoms such as frequency, urgency and dysuria.
- Ureteric obstruction can produce loin pain.
- Microscopic haematuria.

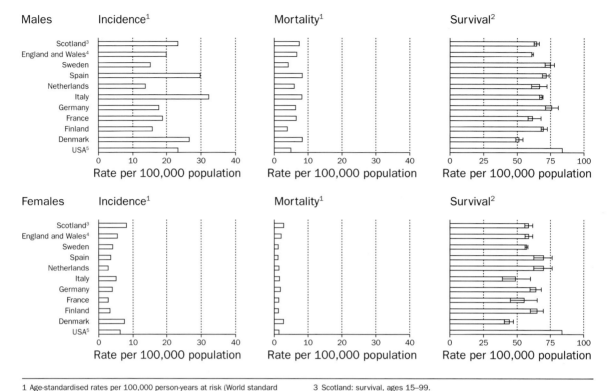

1 Age-standardised rates per 100,000 person-years at risk (World standard population) 1995.
2 Relative survival at 5 years, patients diagnosed 1985–89.

3 Scotland: survival, ages 15–99.
4 England and Wales: incidence 1993; mortality 1995; survival 1986–90 (ages 15–99).
5 USA (SEER, whites): incidence and mortality 1992–96; survival 1989–95.

Figure 4.1 International comparison of incidence, mortality and survival (with 95% CI) all ages, by sex.

Microscopic haematuria in patients with no symptoms

It is almost impossible to attend for a medical without having a dipstick test of urine. There are some guidelines which have been introduced around the country, but, in general, it is rarely worth investigating patients below the age of 40.[3]

Haematuria on testing or on microscopy is found in up to 20% of normal people in the community. If a patient is <40 years, there is between 1.5 and 6% chance of finding a malignancy.[12]

It is said that the use of phase contrast microscopy can distinguish between 'glomerular red cells', which result from glomeru-

lonephritis that is present, and non-glomerular red cells, where bleeding is occurring from the upper urinary tract, other than the glomerulus. Some of these individuals are found to have a uniformly thinned glomerular basement membrane at renal biopsy. This is associated with a very mild proliferative glomerulonephritis, which has a benign prognosis.[13]

Pathology

Inverted papilloma
An inverted papilloma is a benign tumour and presents with haematuria. The tumour is polypoid in appearance and the urothelial cells extend deep into the lamina propria. There is a

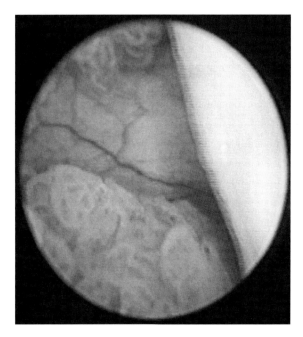

Figure 4.2 Superficial bladder cancer. Retrograde catheter to the right.

lack of mitosis and the tumour is covered by urothelium. The urothelium is of normal thickness and occasionally can be atrophic or hyperplastic. Occasionally, a mucus-containing goblet cell can be seen. An inverted papilloma has a bland cytological appearance, lacking mitotic figures. Dysplasia and mitosis should *not* be identified and if they are present, indicate carcinoma.[14]

Everted papilloma
Occasionally, the papilloma can be called an everted type of papilloma. This is seen in younger individuals. It has a well-ordered appearance, with no more than seven layers of normal appearing urothelial cells and includes a normal basal cell layer. These papillomas are benign.

Nephrogenic adenomata
These are rare lesions and can be regarded as renal rests containing renal collecting tubules.

Very rarely, the malignant counterpart of mesonephric carcinoma is encountered.

Leukoplakia
Leukoplakia of the bladder is a premalignant condition and 20% progress to malignancy.[3] It is regarded as a response to chronic irritation, and is found in patients with long-term catheters, schistosomiasis, and bladder calculi.

Urothelial carcinomas
Urothelial carcinomas are divided into two broad categories: papillary and non-papillary. The appearance of a papillary tumour is that of coral, but when looked at as irrigation fluid flows, it does of course move gently with the motion of the fluid.

WHO classification

The grading system used normally at the World Health Organization (WHO system) includes grades 1–3 and also undifferentiated carcinoma.[15] Grade 1 represents well-differentiated tumours, with very little cellular atypia. Grade 3 is the worst category, but there is still recognisable transitional cell carcinoma.

Bergkvist classification

More recently, Bergkvist proposed a system to give more details. Bergkvist divides stage 2 into 2a and 2b; in 2a the impression of order dominates the system, whereas in 2b there is gross disorder.

A WHO undifferentiated carcinoma is a Bergkvist grade 4.

Risks of progression

Ta tumours have a 4% risk of progression to muscle invasion, whereas T1 tumours have a 30% risk of progression to muscle invasion. Because of this difference, the pathologist will look for invasion of the lamina propria, which is a loose connective tissue below the basement membrane. Smooth muscle fibres are seen in this layer: these are distinct from the muscularis propria. Invasion of the muscularis propria carries the worst prognosis. If Von Brunn's nests are involved, this does not of itself indicate invasion.

Features which predict the worst prognosis include:

- a high grade
- absence or disorganisation of the basement membrane
- invasion below the level of the muscularis mucosa
- deep muscle involvement
- a high number of mitotic figures
- invasion of small vessels, occasionally called microvessel density
- invasion of lymphatic channels
- associated carcinoma – in situ (CIS)
- tumour size
- number of tumours.

Ploidy
Aneuploid tumours have 50% worse survival than diploid tumours at 10 years. The presence of c-*erb*B-2[16] (HER-2 neu), EGFR[17] and p53[18] are associated with invasion. The loss of the Rb gene leads to decreased survival.[19]

Biological markers in superficial bladder cancer

For many years, clinicians have tried to find predictors of both outcome and recurrence. Genes on chromosome 9 are said to act as potential gatekeeper genes. Fradet reviews molecular markers, molecular field changes, cell cycle markers and tumour suppressor genes.[20]

Cyclo-oxygenase-2 (COX) inhibiting drugs have anti-tumour activity in dog and rat models. COX-2 is overexpressed in transitional cell carcinoma and carcinoma in situ, but not in normal urothelium. COX-2 inhibitors may be potential drugs to inhibit bladder tumour behaviour.[21]

It has been shown that a high fluid intake can decrease the risk of bladder cancer in men.[22]

Urothelial dysplasia and carcinoma in situ

Mild, moderate and severe dysplasia have been identified, but reproducibility and interobserver variation have proved a problem. In practice, it is only really severe dysplasia and carcinoma in situ that are important.

CIS (carcinoma in situ)

In CIS, a population of malignant cells replaces the urothelium. This may produce irritative symptoms but may be asymptomatic.

The presence of positive urinary cytology may indicate a particularly aggressive form of transitional cell carcinoma and this test should be carried out on all patients with carcinoma in situ.[23]

Squamous cell carcinoma

Squamous cell carcinoma in many parts of the world is associated with schistosomiasis. Other risk factors may include urinary tract infection and long-term use of an indwelling catheter and stone formation. Chronic irritation may be the factor leading to the development of this carcinoma.

This lesion is normally an ulcerating and invasive tumour. This type of cancer may present in older patients. Partly because of this, the 5-year survival is poor.

CLASSIFICATION OF BLADDER CANCER STAGE

The TNM (tumour, mode, metastasis) staging system for bladder cancer is shown in Table 4.3.

Evaluation of tumour is partly by bimanual palpation. This is essential to evaluate the T stage.

Table 4.3 TNM staging of urinary bladder cancer	
Stage	**Finding**
Ta	Non-invasive papillary
Tis	In situ: 'flat tumour'
T1	Subepithelial connective tissue
T2	Muscularis
T2a	Inner half of muscle
T2b	Outer half of muscle
T3	Beyond muscularis
T3a	Microscopically
T3b	Extravesical mass
T4a	Prostate, uterus, vagina
T4b	Pelvic wall, abdominal wall
N1	Single <2 cm
N2	Single >2 to 5 cm, multiple <5 cm
N3	>5 cm

MANAGEMENT OF EARLY DISEASE

Diagnosis

The commonest form of presentation is that of frank haematuria. Patients presenting with this condition require their upper tracts imaged, usually by an intravenous urogram (IVU), although there is some argument that an ultrasound can be sufficient. An IVU can miss a small renal cell carcinoma. The argument against an ultrasound is that small ureteric lesions can be missed. Often, both modalities are used.

Imaging studies

Intravenous urogram (IVU)
IVU excludes common upper urinary tract tumours and also diagnoses ureteric obstruction caused by bladder tumour.

Ureteric obstruction usually indicates high-stage disease. Hydronephrosis is known to be a prognostic indicator in bladder cancer patients.

More than 90% of those with bilateral hydronephrosis had extravesical extension and this was present in 67% of those with unilateral dilatation. Hydronephrosis does not, however, always indicate extravesical extension and 78% of patients with hydronephrosis were found to have superficial disease in Skinner's 1998 series.[24]

CT scanning
Computed tomography (CT) scanning is insufficiently specific in detecting bladder cancer, particularly at the bladder base. CT scanning is also poor at detecting positive lymph nodes. Mansson indicates that his policy is only to perform CT scanning if there is a palpable large tumour, whether fixed or not, upper urinary tract dilatation, anaemia, or some other sign suggestive of advanced disease.[25]

MR staging
Magnetic resonance (MR) staging is said to be 20% more accurate at staging local disease but cannot distinguish between tumour and post-resection oedema and fibrosis. New MR techniques include three-dimensional sequences and fast dynamic imaging: these may improve staging.[26–28]

PET scanning
Positron emission tomography (PET) scanning may have a place in the future, but at present it has not been shown to be valuable routinely.[29] Choline compounds may be more effective than fluoro deoxy glucose (FDG).

Cystoscopy

Patients with haematuria, or where bladder cancer is suspected should be cystoscoped. Flexible cystoscopy allows identification and biopsy, but usually a rigid cystoscopy is necessary for definitive surgical resection. Small tumours can be removed at a flexible cystoscopy and slightly larger tumours can be excised using laser excision under local anaesthetic. The desire for local anaesthesia must not override the safe excision of the primary tumour.

Small bladder tumours should be excised and sent to pathology using transurethral resection of bladder tumour (TURBT).

Microwave therapy has been used in combination with intravesical mitomycin as an elective approach of conservative treatment for multifocal recurrence of superficial bladder tumour. As yet, although this therapy appears to be efficacious, it remains to be seen whether results are in any way improved over standard electroresection.[30]

particularly with frank haematuria, as soon as possible. Delay in diagnosis and treatment in early disease is important, but may not be critical. It is a greater factor in patients with frank haematuria. In an attempt to streamline treatment, haematuria clinics have been developed. It must be recognised that this is of benefit when frank haematuria is the presenting complaint, but the presence of urgency without haematuria may lead to delay in investigation.[31-35]

Delay in diagnosis

Early diagnosis would be expected to improve outcome and it is prudent to investigate patients,

Transurethral resection of bladder tumour (TURBT)

With the patient under general anaesthetic or spinal anaesthetic, a 26F–28F resectoscope is fit-

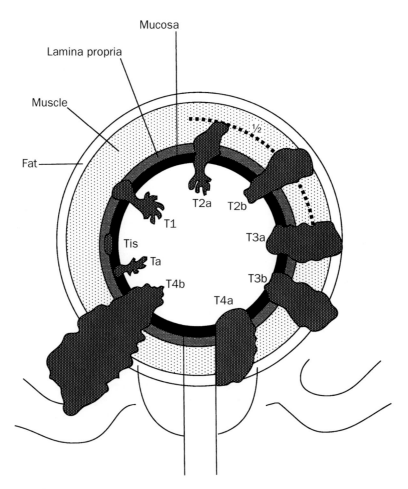

Figure 4.3 T staging of bladder cancer.

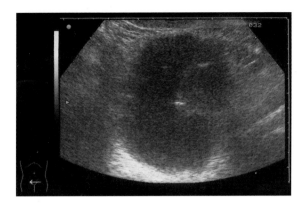

Figure 4.4 Transverse ultrasound image of bladder, demonstrating tumour (seen on the right on left lateral wall).

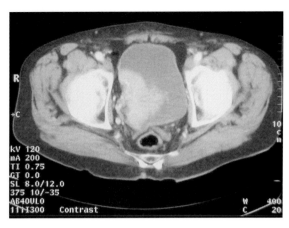

Figure 4.5 Contrast-enhanced CT image of primary bladder cancer arising from right lateral wall of bladder.

ted with a Schmiedt tube, with a 0° lens. This allows the resectoscope to be passed along the urethra under vision and allows identification of any urethral tumours. Prophylactic antibiotics are not necessary routinely but may be used if there is a long resection time. Antibiotics are necessary if there is a proven or suspected urinary tract infection.

Once the urethra has been traversed, a 30° telescope is inserted and the bladder carefully scanned for tumour, in addition to inspecting the area of tumour which is known to be present.

Suprapubic pressure may be used to move the bladder and assist in seeing it all. The patient may be placed head down if it helps visualisation. An experienced operator tends to have a system of inspection, to ensure that all areas are visualised.

Increasingly, surgeons prefer to use a camera system, the camera being attached to the optical portion of the resectoscope. This allows the scope to be manipulated in different directions without the operator having to indulge in contortions. The camera system is particularly useful for looking at the dome of the bladder, near the air bubble.

Once the bladder has been inspected, the Schmiedt tube is replaced by the resectoscope,

with a cutting loop. The tumour is systematically resected and, if possible, the area at the base is sent separately, in formal saline to the pathologist, to allow for identification of invasion.

The irrigation fluid used is 1.5% glycine. It is necessary to change from 0.9% saline, due to the inability of saline to allow electrocautery. A continuous flow resectoscope allows the bladder to be kept half full, which is the optimal situation while resecting. By continually replacing the irrigation fluid, any bleeding which is produced is washed out of the bladder, which allows a faster resection. This is particularly important in more elderly or frail patients.

Diathermy of any bleeding vessels is carried out either with the loop, or if no discrete vessels are seen, cauterisation with a rolly ball electrode.

The bladder should be washed out with an Ellik evacuator. The principle here is to introduce maximum turbulence within the bladder and ensure that small bladder biopsies do not linger in the bladder or get stuck in diverticula. Normal saline is generally used and the specimen retrieved and sent to pathology. Sterile water can also be used to wash out the bladder and this has the additional feature of lysing cancer cells which may still be present in the

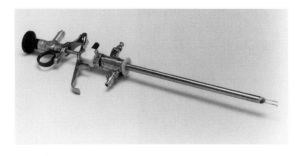

Figure 4.6 Standard resectoscope with working electrocautery element (loop) to the right.

bladder. It is essential to remember that water is toxic if absorbed in any quantity, and may be contraindicated if it is thought that there is a significant risk of absorption. This would produce haemolysis and would mimic a transurethral resection of prostate (TURP) syndrome.

At this stage, the surgeon ensures that bleeding is minimal. The resectoscope is removed and further lubrication inserted into the urethra, before insertion of a 20–22F three-way catheter. If the bleeding is minimal, then postoperative irrigation is unnecessary and the irrigation channel can be spigotted. It does, however, allow the bladder to be lavaged. It is prudent to inspect the effluent in the recovery area before leaving operating theatre, since a bladder washout in the early stages avoids the patient having to be taken back to the operating theatre at a later time.

If it is a policy, then a chemotherapeutic instillation of mitomycin may be given at this stage.

With the anaesthetist's permission, an analgesic suppository such as diclofenac (Voltarol) is inserted.

At the beginning and at the end of any resection, an examination under anaesthesia (EUA) is carried out and the clinical staging of the tumour recorded.

During resection, care should be taken that large biopsies are taken, which minimises any heat artifact in the tissues.

Occasionally, tumours are seen emanating from the ureteric orifice and these can be easily resected. Although this can lead to reflux, it is possible to cure these tumours by resection; but, of course, careful surveillance is necessary.

A ureteric stent can be inserted if there is any concern about the ureteric continuity with the bladder.

Occasionally, tumours can be seen in bladder diverticula. The wall of the diverticulum is thin and easily perforated. It may be possible to carefully resect tumour in a diverticulum. When we have our concerns about going into deeper tissues, then a partial cystectomy or total cystectomy may be indicated. Some authorities would recommend chemotherapy or radiotherapy in this situation.

Bladder perforation
Occasionally, the integrity of the bladder wall is compromised and the patient may extravasate fluid. This can be indicated by some localised discomfort; ensure that any irrigation is not carried out at high pressure in these circumstances and manage the patient by giving diuretics and curtailing the irrigation.

It is prudent to give antibiotics in these circumstances. Any perforation into the peritoneal cavity should be monitored with close concern. If there is doubt, a cystogram may show fluid entering the peritoneal cavity. It is better to risk an unnecessary laparotomy, if any doubt remains, as the perforation can easily be sutured and a drain inserted.

Another indication for laparotomy is severe pain, with drainage of the surrounding tissue and suture of any perforation noted.

It has become fashionable to use disposable Ellik evacuators and the advantage of these is that the specimen can be sent in the evacuator to the Pathology Department without requiring handling.

It is prudent to change the evacuating fluid over a period of time, since constant use of an evacuator may lead to a build up of endotoxin and bacteria.

In many departments, a broad-spectrum antibiotic is given routinely for TURBT.

Urinary cytology is not generally helpful at

the time of cystoscopy and if it is to be carried out, it should be carried out either prior to cystoscopy, or several weeks after the cystoscopy.

It is standard practice to remove the tumour endoscopically wherever possible. Many authorities would suggest biopsies of the 'normal bladder epithelium': this can be either a near and far biopsy, or four-quadrant biopsies.

> It should be remembered that the number of biopsies increases the work of the pathologist and may in fact hinder the presentation of information, by camouflaging results of greater significance.

With one bladder tumour of low mitotic appearance, it is usually sufficient to arrange for a further check cystoscopy in 3 months' time.

Laser and microwave energy

Lasers can be used to treat bladder tumours. The Nd:YAG (neodymium:yttrium–aluminium–garnet) laser penetrates only to a depth of 3–5 mm. It is mainly of use for tissue coagulation. Lasers are said to have a lower risk of tumour dissemination, but the evidence is not strong. Lasers also have very controlled areas of action; they do not allow biopsies to be taken, since the tumour is vaporised. The main disadvantage is the relatively high cost. It is possible to carry out limited treatment under local anaesthetic, making the technique suitable for flexible cytoscopy. The lack of bleeding allows treatment in patients on anticoagulants.

Lasers may be used with haematoporphyrin derivative (HPD) as photodynamic therapy. The individual may be sensitised to the HPD, and it usually cannot be administered more than once.

Microwave therapy has been used in combination with intravesical mitomycin as an elective approach of conservative treatment for multifocal recurrence of superficial bladder tumour. As yet, although it appears to be efficacious, it remains to be seen whether results are in any way improved over standard electroresection.[36]

Follow-up of superficial disease

A programme of follow-up – of so-called check cystoscopy – is appropriate for Ta and T1 disease. There is a high risk of recurrence, but even in those whose disease behaves more benignly, follow-up is indicated for life. At more than 5 years, some clinicians change from endoscopic monitoring to cytology and to tests such as BTA™.[37] Endoscopy is the safest option in terms of tumour control, especially if the patient will tolerate flexible cystoscopy (the risks of recurrence are listed in Table 4.4).

Radiotherapy in superficial bladder disease

Radiotherapy is not successful in controlling superficial disease, and there are high recurrence rates.[38] It can, however, prevent recurrence in 15% of patients, with G3 T1 lesions.[39]

Some authorities would recommend the instillation of antimitotic drugs such as mitomycin at the time of primary resection. This undoubtedly reduces the recurrence rate, but has not been shown to increase survival.

> Occasionally, the patient will present with numerous tumours and these must all be removed

It is important to wash the bladder out carefully, to avoid implantation of cells. Occasionally, superficial disease presents, with so many tumours studded over the bladder that the urologist is unable to control these at interval cystoscopies (Table 4.4). If these are well-differentiated tumours, the use of mitomycin or epirubicin is indicated. If this medication fails to control the number of recurrent bladder tumours, then a fit patient should be offered cystectomy.

Occasionally, tumours have a high-grade appearance under microscopy, i.e. G3 tumours. These are the tumours to be watched carefully. Some authorities would suggest very early radiotherapy for these tumours and a urologist might elect for a very early cystectomy.[41,42]

Table 4.4 Risk of recurrence (from Reading et al[40])			
Risk category	No. of tumours	First cytoscopy	1-year recurrence free
Good	Solitary	No recurrence	75%
Moderate	Solitary	Recurrence	50%
	Multiple	No recurrence	
Poor	Multiple	Recurrence	20%

Intravesical therapy

Thiotepa (triethylenethiophosphoramide), an alkylating agent, was the first intravesical agent used in the treatment of bladder cancer. It produces tumour remission in 35% of patients with superficial bladder tumours but is not so effective in CIS. It is absorbed through the bladder endothelium and can cause myelosuppression in up to 20% of patients, requiring monitoring of white cell counts before each treatment.[3]

Mitomycin C is an antibiotic. It has a higher molecular weight than thiotepa, but about 1% is absorbed. It can cause chemical cystitis, skin rashes and calcification of the bladder wall. The chemical cystitis can lead to contraction of the bladder.[3]

Doxorubicin (adriamycin) is also an antibiotic: it is minimally absorbed due to its high molecular weight. It can cause skin rashes and is not so popular as mitomycin c.[43]

Epirubicin is a derivative of the above and has reduced toxicity, being better tolerated.[44]

BCG

BCG (bacille Calmette-Guérin) is an attenuated strain of *Mycobacterium bovis*. There are a number of strains available and all of them emanate from the original strain at the Pasteur Institute. Strains include Pasteur, Tice, Connaught and Evans. Viability is usually quoted in colony-forming units.

The BCG is administered intravesically, in weekly instillations over a period of 6 weeks. It must not be given to immunocompromised patients or after a traumatic catheterisation.

No additional benefit is seen when it is given intradermally. It is thought to work by stimulating immune mechanisms and must adhere to the bladder tumour. It can be very effective in tumours which have been incompletely resected, and about 58% are said to respond. Its main use is in CIS and complete responses (CR) are of the order of 70%.[45]

Side effects
These include

- bladder irritability
- granulomatous prostatitis
- BCGosis – a systemic illness mimicking tuberculosis.

Fever persisting for more than 48 hours after BCG treatment should be treated with isoniazid (300 mg daily) with pyridoxine (50 mg daily).

Where fever is high or more protracted, rifampicin (600 mg daily) should be added. It is prudent to seek the help of a physician skilled in the management of tuberculosis. A 6-month course of therapy is generally indicated in these severe cases.

Other biological agents

Other agents such as interferon, especially alpha-2b, and interleukin-2 have been tried, but no agent has achieved popularity.[46–48]

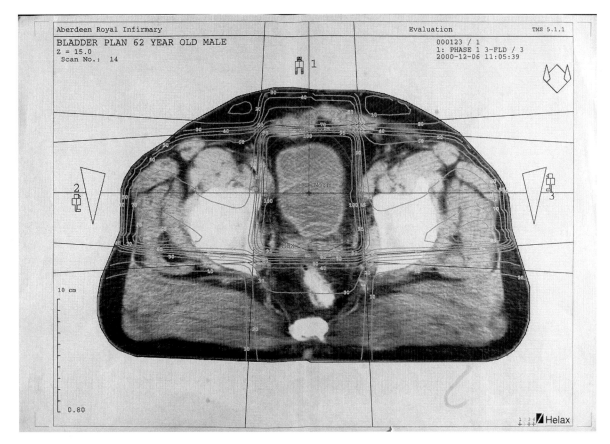

Figure 4.7 Bladder cancer radiotherapy plan.

MUSCLE INVASIVE DISEASE

External beam radiotherapy for muscle invasive disease

Cystectomy has always been claimed as the treatment of choice in dealing with muscle invasive disease. Radiotherapists may claim with some justification that they are not always offered the same type of patient, their patients being generally less fit and less able to withstand surgery.

We know that the survival at 5 years is about 30–40% in patients with T2 tumours and between 5 and 20% in patients with T3 and T4 tumours.

Local control is achieved by a dose of 60 Gy given in 30 fractions, over 6 weeks.

In an attempt to achieve bladder preservation, extensive local resection has been combined with radiotherapy. Although results following radiotherapy have been poorer than results reported from cystectomy, at least 50% of patients may require salvage cystectomy.[49]

A typical plan for radiotherapy is shown in Figure 4.8

Bladder-sparing techniques

Herr and his colleagues reported 70% of patients preserving their bladder, where extensive local resection was combined with radiation therapy. They reported a 5-year survival rate of 80%.

The factors which influence survival and local recurrence are T stage, tumour grade, pretreatment haemoglobin levels, whether or not there is tumour left after TURBT and evidence of ureteric obstruction.

Many centres in North America are now offering combined radiation and chemotherapy for bladder-sparing treatment.[50,51]

PATIENTS WITH HIGH-GRADE LESIONS BEING PREPARED FOR CYSTECTOMY

The risk of urethral recurrence after cystoprostatectomy is between 5 and 15%. The classical risk factors were CIS of the bladder, tumour multifocality, tumour at the bladder neck, upper tract tumour and prostatic involvement.[52–54]

> It has been found that the incidence of urethral recurrence increases greatly if there is stromal invasion of the prostate, increasing from 25% if there is ductal involvement only, to 64%.[55]

Skinner and his colleagues[56] suggest that ileum connected to urethra may protect the urethra from recurrent transitional cell carcinoma, but further information of this is awaited.

> At present, it is recommended that frozen-section biopsies be taken of the urethra if an orthotopic reconstruction is being considered.[56]

MANAGEMENT OF THE RETAINED URETHRA AFTER CYSTECTOMY

Although the prostatic and penile urethra are rarely removed at cystectomy, they are at risk of transitional cell carcinoma.

Follow up must involve a high index of suspicion. The native urethra can be cystoscoped and/or urethral washings can be taken for cytology. Certainly if there is a bloody urethral discharge, it is imperative that this is done, but this may be too late to deal with the tumour. At this stage, if tumour is found, a urethrectomy is indicated, assuming there is no evidence of any secondary disease.

The technique involves incision through the perineum, which allows the urethra to be removed and the penis inverted. A catheter through the urethra allows the urethra to be pulled down and the penis is turned inside out.

URINARY DIVERSION

Cystectomy is often the best way of removing an organ that may have one obvious focus of tumour but has also the potential to develop further tumours. The patient may be offered the choice between a continent diversion and an ileal conduit which is of course not continent.

Factors deciding the optimal method for urinary tract reconstruction on a patient undergoing cystectomy are:

- age
- nodal status
- risk of urethral recurrence
- previous pelvic radiation
- renal function
- physical status
- psychological functioning.[57]

Radical cystectomy and urinary diversion (OPCS code M3400, cystectomy M344, standard ileal conduit M191, construction of continent reservoir M198b)

This technique remains the most common curative treatment but requires a reasonably fit patient.

Radical cystectomy remains one of the most effective methods of control of invasive bladder cancer.

The construction of an ileal conduit remains a tried and tested method of urinary diversion. One of the earliest descriptions was by Bricker.[58]

Increasingly, it is important that this procedure is discussed in depth with the patient, to weigh up all the disadvantages. In younger patients, who are highly motivated, a discussion of other techniques of diversion should be undertaken. Also, the presence of a stoma may have difficulties for certain religions and must be discussed with patients.

Patients may have had radiotherapy to their bladder and, where local recurrence has taken place, the rather clumsy term of salvage cystectomy has been coined.

Indications

- flat in-situ transitional cell carcinoma of bladder usually where BCG therapy has failed (T1b)
- multiple papillary tumours of bladder uncontrolled by endoscopic means (Ta, T1)
- invasive transitional cell carcinoma (TCC) of bladder (T2, T3)
- bladder TCC invading the prostate (T4a)
- squamous carcinoma of the bladder
- sarcoma of the bladder.

This is a major procedure and the patient must be assessed for fitness, independent of age.

Preoperative preparation

An IVU is necessary to exclude widespread TCC in ureters.

Exclude metastatic disease by staging:

- chest X-ray
- bone scan
- CT of pelvis and abdomen.

Blood tests

- Haemoglobin (Hb) and full blood count (FBC)
- Urea and electrolytes
- Liver function tests.

Other tests

- Electrocardiography (ECG).
- Echocardiography (where indicated by significant cardiac disease).

Cross-match

Four units of packed cells are cross-matched.

Heparin

Low molecular weight heparin (5000 units subcutaneously) preoperatively on the day before surgery until the patient is ambulant. Anti-thrombogenic stockings are applied.

Operating theatre

An operating time of at least 4 hours is booked. Two assistants must be free, at least one of whom is experienced.

Consent

Radical cystectomy implies pelvic lymphadenectomy of the iliac and obturator nodes.

In the male, the bladder is removed en bloc, along with the pelvic peritoneum, ureteric remnants, prostate and seminal testicles and a small piece of membranous urethra.

In the female, the uterus, ovaries, fallopian tubes, vaginal vault and urethra are removed. This is discussed in full, but it means they will not need cervical smears.

Sexual function is usually lost in both sexes.

Admission

The patient is brought into the ward 2 days prior to surgery and started on a low-residue diet.

The stoma nurse, or similar counsellor, is booked to discuss the practical aspects of the stoma and show the patient the fitting of the appliance. The patient is shown how to change this and, after discussion, the site for the stoma is chosen below the belt line, paying particular attention to skin folds and avoiding previous scars. This site is marked with an indelible skin pencil.

On the day prior to surgery, the patient is patch-tested for iodine. The patient is only permitted clear fluids to drink.

A bowel cleaning solution (Picolax sachets) is given at 10 a.m. and again at 2 p.m. If there is no result, a Microlax enema (sodium citrate) can then be given, or a high phosphate enema, if the patient has not opened their bowels for several days. If the patient is frail, urea and electrolytes may be checked on the morning of surgery to identify hypokalaemia. An intravenous infusion may be requested overnight prior to surgery.

Where high dependency unit (HDU) facilities are available, epidural analgesia may be beneficial and may be mandatory if the patient has pulmonary disease. The pain team discuss analgesics. The physiotherapist instructs the patient on breathing and leg exercises.

Surgical anatomy of the bladder

The fundus of the bladder lies behind the symphysis pubis. The median umbilical ligament may join the bladder to the umbilicus. This is the remains of the urachus. The blood supply of the bladder comes from the superior and inferior vesical arteries. There can occasionally be small branches from the inferior epigastric artery. Drainage is through the vesical plexus, which joins with the prostatic plexus in the male and drains into the internal iliac veins.

Patient position

The operation is performed under general anaesthetic with muscle relaxation. The patient is placed supine, and the presence of a small sandbag behind the lumbar spine aids vision within the pelvis.

In view of the occasional high blood loss, many anaesthetists insert a central venous pressure line and, where the patient is unfit, an arterial line. Where the patient is unfit, it is also prudent to ensure that there is an intensive therapy unit (ITU) bed available. Compression boots are applied in the operating theatre.

Instruments

- Laparotomy crate/major general set
- Doyen's bowel clamps (or similar non-crushing clamps)
- Bowel tray
- Ring retractor (Turner-Warwick)
- Diathermy
- Wallace drain introducer
- McDougall's right- and left-angle clamps
- Potts right-angle scissors.

Procedure

The antibiotics, Augmentin (co-amoxiclav) and metronidazole are given intravenously soon after anaesthetic induction.

The patient is catheterised with a 16-French (16F) Foley catheter and the bladder drained. The patient is prepared using an iodine skin preparation, draped exposing the abdomen from xiphisternum to pelvis. The cross marking the prepared site for the conduit is then transfixed with a silk suture, so that the site of the conduit does not become obliterated during the operation. The vagina is packed with an iodine-soaked swab.

Incision

A standard midline incision is used, skirting the umbilicus. This must avoid the projected stoma site and allow plenty of room, for fitting of an appliance.

It is feasible to do a transverse abdominal incision, but the disadvantage with this approach is that it is difficult to free up the greater omentum if it is stuck in the higher part of the abdomen. For this reason, I prefer a midline incision.

Division of the attachments of the rectus abdominis to the pelvic line, as originally described by Richard Turner-Warwick, aids exposure.

Approach

The abdomen is opened. Nowadays, the patient will have previously had an abdominal and a pelvic CAT scan, but it is sensible just to check that no large lesion has been missed in the liver. At this stage, it is also easy to free the greater omentum.

Two dry packs are used to retract the abdominal contents and a ring retractor is then placed in position.

The first approach is to open the retroperitoneal space and expose each obturator fossa in turn. Any lymph nodes are excised and sent in separate jars to Pathology.

The lymph nodes are dissected, taking all tissue medial to the genitofemoral nerve off the iliopsoas muscle and the external iliac vessels, including the fat pad at the inguinal ligament. The lymph node (Cloquet's node) at the femoral canal is also removed. The obturator nodes are removed and they lie between the external and internal iliac vessels.

At this stage, it is useful to expose the ureters and place sloops around each.

The bladder can then gradually be mobilised. At this stage, it is possible to decide whether the bladder can be removed.

If the scans are accurate, it is rare that this decision has to be reversed. Once this decision is made, the ureters can be divided at leisure. I place 2.0 Vicryl (polyglactin 910) sutures around each distal end of the ureter and leave long tails. This is to allow the ureters to dilate, stops urine washing into the peritoneal cavity and the long tails allow easy identification at a later stage.

The vasa deferentes (or the round ligaments in females) are divided bilaterally (to avoid small bowel strangulation).

The pedicles of the bladder can be divided, using a mixture of sharp and blunt dissection and automatic clips. The superior and inferior vesical arteries carry out most of the blood supply.

The pelvic fascia may be opened on either side of the bladder and Santorini's venous plexus divided, as one would with a radical prostatectomy. This can allow much easier mobilisation of the bladder and prostate.

The parietal peritoneum over the bladder should be removed to allow the small bowel ultimately to fall into the pelvic cavity. Failure to do this can lead to a pyopelvis.

The bladder is removed and any obvious bleeding points diathermied or tied.

A dry pack is then placed in the pelvis and attention is then turned to fashioning the ileal conduit.

The appendix is identified and, because continent diversion is not being used, there is still a strong argument for removing the appendix, since appendicitis in patients with an ileal conduit can be very difficult to diagnose.

Ileal conduit

The terminal ileum is then identified and a portion of ileum is isolated, avoiding the terminal 25 cm of terminal ileum, which is where bowel salts are reabsorbed. The distance can be measured. The small bowel is transilluminated using a satellite lamp at right angles to the bowel.

The small bowel is divided between noncrushing Doyen's clamps. At this stage, I find it very helpful to identify the terminal end of the conduit, by marking it with a long Vicryl suture. It is remarkably easy to get these ends reversed during a longer procedure, and identification at this stage avoids difficulties later on.

The small bowel is re-anastomosed using controlled release 3.0 Nurolon (polymide 6 braided nonabsorbable, Ethicon) sutures and the window of the mesentery is repaired using interrupted absorbable sutures (2/0 Vicryl). In most cases, the small bowel sits better in an inferior position, below the anastomosis.

A Bachaus towel clip can be used to approximate the Doyen's clamps while the anastomosis is performed.

The distal ends of the ureters can then be identified using the long tags suture and tunnels are made so that the created gap in the posterior layer of the peritoneum acts as a window through which the ureters are drawn. The left ureter is drawn through the sigmoid mesocolon. Once again the tags of silk may be used to assist this.

The conduit is irrigated with a normal saline solution, ensuring that any remaining debris is removed.

The ends of the ureters are then spatulated and the terminal ends of Vicryl sutures can be held together until the anastomosis is partially fashioned. At this stage, size 6F infant feeding tubes are passed into each ureter and drawn through the conduit. The cap on the infant feeding tube is taken off the left one (shorter tube, shorter number of letters) and I found that a 3.0 Vicryl suture placed through the ureter, but not through its maximum circumference, anchors the tube. The suture must of course be absorbable. Alternatively, an 8F single J stent may be used and does not need suturing. I use the method described by Wallace, and usually a Wallace 1. There is an argument for the Bricker technique, which is said to reduce reflux and possible tumour recurrence.

The anastomosis is then completed. At this stage, the integrity of the anastomosis is tested using 50 ml of saline, injected gently with a bladder tip syringe into the distal end of the conduit. Any small leaks are sutured.

Fashioning of the stoma

The Vicryl stitch on the skin, at the site of the stoma, is lifted. This allows an easy excision of a circular area of skin. A tract is then fashioned through the muscle layers (preferably through rectus abdominis to avoid parastomal hernias) into the abdomen, and the distal end of the conduit is drawn through the skin. Care must be taken that there is no obstruction at this point.

It is imperative that there is no tension on this anastomosis. If there is any tension or marked ischaemia, then a new conduit must be fashioned. The ends of the conduit are turned back on themselves, with four sutures, 4.0 Dexon (Davis and Geck) at each corner, securing the distal end to the lower proximal area, thus everting the stoma.

The anastomosis can then be dropped back into the retroperitoneum, but at this stage the omentum is drawn down and wrapped around this area to allow for revascularisation.

Any redundant omentum is also placed near the small bowel anastomosis.

At this point, attention is then turned to the pelvis again. Any residual bleeders can be dealt with at leisure.

Closure
I close with two 20F Wallace drains (Robinson drainage system), brought out through separate stab incisions on each iliac fossa, the drains being secured with a suture of 2.0 silk. One drain is led up to the area of the conduit and the other drain is led down into the pelvis.

The urethral catheter has of course been divided when the urethra was divided and, unless urethrectomy has been carried out, nothing further need be done at this point.

I close with No. 1 PDS suture with a blunt taper point needle, taking all layers.

Skin closure is a matter of choice, but I think there is a strong argument for using skin staples, since the operation is already long enough. A stoma bag is applied over the conduit.

Postoperative care
The patient's vital signs are monitored and, in particular, the urine output is charted. A small degree of haematuria is to be expected.

The drains are removed when they stop draining and, where a nasogastric tube has been inserted, the patient may be given 15–30 ml of fluid hourly after 6–8 hours.

Specific complications
Early
- Urinary leakage

- Lymphatic leakage
- Ileus.

Late (after 6 weeks)
- Recurrent urinary tract infection (UTI)
- Parastomal hernia
- Ureteric strictures – probably ischaemic
- Stomal infarction – ischaemic
- Stomal retraction
- Stomal stricture
- Acidosis
- Bilateral hydronephrosis
- Renal stone.

Key points
Patient selection is paramount
ITU/HDU bed available *if needed*
The conduit must be well vascularised
The conduit must not be constricted at the abdominal wall

An experienced team of nursing staff, theatre staff must be available, in addition to an experienced anaesthetist and an experienced operator.

PRINCIPLES OF CONTINENT RECONSTRUCTION

New bladders require the following characteristics:

1. adequate potential volumes
2. low pressure
3. minimal or no absorption characteristics
4. good reservoir emptying
5. no reflux problems.

Continence mechanisms

These are generally twofold: nipple valves and flap valves.

Nipple valves
The technique involves the contents of the reservoir compressing the nipple, which is a length of tissue within the reservoir.[3]

Flap valves
This technique requires pressure within the reservoir to press upon the distal end of the ureter.

Continent diversionz

- Many patients want a reservoir which is continent and which is accessed by catheterisation.
- Bowel segments, usually constructed by the use of small bowel are detubularised and fashioned into a neobladder or pouch after methods described by Koch or Studer.
- Various continence mechanisms are described. The Mitrofanoff principle describes the use of the appendix, which can be catheterised at will.
- The bowel may be fashioned into a continent port if the appendix is not suitable or is absent.
- Where the patient's own urethra is used, the term orthotopic is used.

These methods of diversion are more difficult and time-consuming than ileal conduit surface diversions and are the province of a specialist. Patients must be advised that often multiple operations are necessary, and they are not for patients who are unfit.

CONTINENT URINARY DIVERSION

Uretero-sigmoid diversion

Technical aspects
The use of ureteric stenting is generally preferred and the rectal tube is inserted. This can be removed after a gastrografin enema has demonstrated the integrity of the anastomosis.

Many patients find a rectal tube to be inserted at night to be of benefit, and this is certainly necessary in those who have electrolyte problems.[3]

Kock developed a technique and called it augmented valved rectum; this technique uses a proximally intussuscepted sigmoid colon to confine the urine to a smaller area.[59]

There are other variations of this technique, i.e. a hemi-Kock procedure, with valved rectum. This was developed where the ureters were too dilated to bring them into the intussuscepted sigmoid. Skinner modified this technique to head to the rectum after sigmoid intussusception.

A further variation of ureterosigmoidoscopy is that of the sigma rectum pouch or MAINZ II pouch.[60]

Orthotopic voiding diversions

Orthotopic means occupying the normal position in the body: this technique therefore implies the use of the patient's normal urethra. Initially, this was confined to male patients, but now increasingly, females are being offered this procedure.

It is important that patients have urethral biopsies, as described elsewhere in this chapter. All patients need to be warned that it may be necessary for them to carry out intermittent self-catheterisation.

Surgical procedures

Camey II operation – procedure
A 65 cm length of ileum is isolated and the continuity of the gut restored. The bowel is allowed to fall down, without tension to the urethra, and then opened throughout its length, with the exception of the portion which is selected to form the urethral anastomosis. It is then sutured back upon itself and the ureters are implanted to the lateral horns of the U, so created using ureteric stents. The new bladder is also drained by a urethral catheter. The complications in this procedure include stenosis of the urethral and ureteric anastomosis. A variation of the Camey technique is that of the ileal neobladder.[61] This variation creates a U-shaped flap, which becomes a new bladder neck.

Hemi-Kock pouch

This procedure, described by Ghoneim in 1987, is similar to an orthotopic hemi-Kock, but it leaves a smaller hole, patent to be used for the anastomosis. There is doubt as to the best way of draining the ureter, whether it should be through double JJ stents, whose lower end is within the neobladder or single J stents brought out through the reservoir to the surface, thus diverting urine from the pouch.

Studer pouch

This was described by Studer and his colleagues as a way of creating a low-pressure bladder. It appears to be a simple, reliable procedure.

Procedure

A 65 cm ileal segment length is isolated and the continuity of the bowel restored. The proximal 25 cm of the ileum are left intact, and this is the portion used for ureteric anastomosis. The distal 40 cm or so is opened along the mesenteric border and folded back upon itself. Stents from the ureters are brought out through the most distal portion of the bowel and the most dependent portion is anastomosed through the urethra, with six urethral sutures, having previously inserted a Foley catheter through the opening in the ileum.

Studer maintains that the intact 20 cm proximal ileal limb prevents or substantially reduces reflux.

Colonic pouches

There is a variety of colonic pouches which are really beyond the remit of this volume. The MAINZ pouch uses the caecum and the distal ileum. The ileocolonic pouch (Le-Bag) is a modification of the MAINZ pouch.

The right colon pouch is a variation that uses the entire right colon. In a similar fashion, the sigmoid colon has been used, as has the stomach.

Continent diversions requiring self-catheterisation

These pouches are used where the native urethra is not felt to be satisfactory. A catheterising port is brought out either at the umbilicus or in the lower quadrant of the abdomen. This bladder site has the advantage of being below the 'bikini' line.

The appendix is frequently used as a new urethra. The other continence mechanism, which is of major interest, is the use of the tapered terminal ileum and ileocaecal valve. These techniques can be adapted to the various pouches which have been described, such as the Kock pouch, MAINZ pouch and the all the various right colonic pouches and all the reservations of the continence caecal reservoir, such as the UCLA pouch, the Duke pouch and the Le Bag.

Frequent self-catheterisation causes trauma to the new urethra. The Indiana pouch is a method of buttressing the ileocaecal valve and using an ileal patch, which should address this factor.[62,63]

Complications of continent urinary diversion

- Death
- Stenosis of stoma
- Prolapse of continence nipple
- Stone formation in pouch
- Metabolic complications
- Urinary infection
- Excess mucus production
- Rupture of pouch.

Abol-Enein and Ghoneim have produced an interesting variation of the serous-lined extramural tunnel. This is an elegant technique which has produced good short-term results.[64,65]

Quality of life following different types of urinary diversion

Mansson & Mansson reviewed the quality of life following different types of diversion. They conclude that quality of life measurement is still in its infancy, despite the many instruments in use; an operation that is optional for a 50-year-old patient, may not be appropriate for a 75-year-old patient.[66]

PATIENT COMMUNICATION IN BLADDER CANCER

In Newcastle a clinical nurse specialist conducted an analysis of the information needs of patients with bladder cancer.[67] The following are the key findings, some of which echo the needs of cancer patients in general:

- Although other staff play an important role in providing information, the urologist is regarded as 'the specialist' who therefore bears the main responsibility for talking with patients and providing the information that they need.
- The diagnosis is a shock for most patients, which prevents them from hearing or understanding much of the information given to them at the time of diagnosis. If patients are to assimilate the information they need, it will need to be repeated on other more appropriate occasions.
- Patients are not 'fully informed' if the information they have been given has not been received or has been misunderstood.
- Most patients want to know 'the whole truth', but this may need to be explained over time and at a pace that matches the patient's ability to cope.
- Nurses, data managers and non-medical staff are perceived by patients as providing unbiased views and therefore compliment what the specialist has said.
- Inaccurate or incomplete information usually does more harm than good.
- Patients with G1 Ta, T1 bladder cancer need just as much information as those with more advanced cancer.
- Written information in the form of a series of separate leaflets rather than one comprehensive booklet or video is an essential addition to personal discussion.
- The need for information does not stop with discharge from hospital following TUR or cystectomy.
- 'We will remove your bladder and rebuild it with part of the bowel' is not an adequate description of what will happen.
- Being offered a choice of treatment disturbs some patients, but most understand, appreciate and regard as essential an explanation of all treatment options.
- The relationship with data managers or research nurses is appreciated by trial patients as a help for them in coping with their cancer.

Quality-of-life questionnaires are often appreciated by patients as an expression of concern for them as a person rather than as a disease.

TREATMENT OF ADVANCED DISEASE

Chemotherapy can produce worthwhile responses and M-VAC (a regimen of methotrexate, vinblastine, doxorubicin and cisplatin) is most commonly used. Akaza reviews advances in chemotherapy of invasive bladder cancer. It is doubted that there are any regimens which are an improvement on M-VAC, but this may be disputed.[68]

Sylvester & Sternberg[69] reviewed the role of adjuvant combination chemotherapy after cystectomy in locally advanced bladder cancer. They analysed many of the published studies and in their critique cite much evidence. They found too much emphasis was put on subgroup analysis and underpowered trials and generally felt that many of the studies have major methodological problems and even mention contradictory claims in dealing with results. They also mention the early stopping of trials, confusing analysis, confusing terminology and questionable conclusions.

At present, an EORTC study has been set up to examine survival after immediate chemotherapy, after cystectomy versus chemotherapy at relapse. It is only by supporting large studies that reliable results will be obtained.[69]

Second-line chemotherapy in advanced bladder cancer

Although the M-VAC regimen remains the gold standard, this may be shifting due to early diagnosis. M-VAC toxicity may be severe and a median survival duration is only 13 months. Only 15% of patients with metastases in visceral sites achieve long-term survival and there have therefore been a number of trials looking at taxanes, gemcitabine and new antifolates, such as trimetrexate and piritrexim.[70]

PROGNOSTIC FACTORS IN BLADDER CANCER

- Stage
- Grade
- DNA ploidy
- p53 tumour-suppressor gene
- Retinoblastoma gene
- E cadherin
- Epidermal growth factor receptor (EGFR)
- Angiogenesis
- Presence of CIS
- Multifocality
- Frequency of recurrence.

A CASE HISTORY OF BLADDER CANCER
(patient permission obtained)

A 60-year-old salesman originally presented some 10 years ago, with a poor urinary stream, frequency and nocturia, rising twice or three times nightly. He had slight dribbling and a feeling of incomplete emptying.

On examination he had a rather tight foreskin and his prostate felt clinically enlarged. He had some pain in his right hip and a plain X-ray confirmed the presence of osteoarthritis. A urinary flow test confirmed a poor stream (Q_{max} = 5.9, voided volume = 280 ml) and a TURP was carried out. About 50 g of prostate were removed and he made an uneventful recovery. The histology of his prostate showed nodular hyperplasia but, in addition, there were three small foci of well-differentiated adenocarcinoma. His prostate-specific antigen (PSA) postoperatively was 5.3.

He was reviewed at 6 monthly intervals, and his PSA dropped to 3.7. He began to develop frequency and no infection was found in his urine. Antibiotic therapy had produced no effect.

A further cystoscopy showed irregularity of his prostate. A further prostatic biopsy was carried out and his histology showed benign hyperplasia; however, surprisingly, there were areas of transitional cell carcinoma noted. The lesion exhibited moderate atypia.

His bladder had been inspected on both occasions and no abnormality had been seen. He had bilateral cough impulses and had bilateral hernias repaired without difficulty by another surgeon.

On his next check cystoscopy there appeared to be a tiny recurrence on the prostatic bed and there was an area in the bladder which looked abnormal. This was biopsied. This showed that there was infiltration by poorly differentiated transitional cell carcinoma, grade 3, and was seen to infiltrate the lamina propria (T4a).

The patient was given a course of radiotherapy (64 Gy in 32 fractions), since he did not wish to have cystectomy.

A further check cystoscopy showed infiltration of the bladder base, by poorly differentiated carcinoma, which was within the subepithelial connective tissue, but no muscular areas or propria was included within the specimen.

On receipt of this biopsy, a further discussion was undertaken with the patient. He finally agreed to have a cystoprostatectomy and ileal conduit. He declined a reconstructive procedure. His operation proceeded without incident. Postoperatively he had some discomfort rectally and responded to a foam preparation of steroids administered per rectum. Histology showed superficially invasive grade 3 transitional cell carcinoma, which was widespread, but the tumour was confined to the submucosal fibroconnective tissue. The resection margins were clear. The prostate contained several foci of well-differentiated invasive prostatic adenocarcinoma (Gleason 3 + 2 = 5). His PSA has remained at less than 0.1. Subsequent urea and electrolytes were normal and routine IVUs carried out at 1–2 yearly intervals have shown no upper tract hydronephrosis or tumour, for 8 years.

REFERENCES

1. Kipling R. In: The Works of Rudyard Kipling. History of England. The Glory of the Garden, 1911. London: The Wordsworth Poetry Library, 1994

2. Rehn L. Blasengeschwulste bei Fuchsin-Arbeitern. Arch Klin Chir 1895; 50:588–600

3. Messing EM, Catalona W. In: Campbell's urology, 7th edn, Walsh P, Retik A, Vaughan ED, Wein A (eds). Philadelphia: WB Saunders, 1997

4. Parkin DM, Whelan SL, Ferlay J, Raymond L, Young J (eds). Cancer incidence in five continents, Vol. VII. IARC Scientific Publications No. 143. Lyon: International Agency for Research on Cancer, 1997

5. Vineis P, Esteve J, Hartge P. Effects of timing and type of tobacco in cigarette-induced bladder cancer. Cancer Res 1998; 48:3849–3852

6. Cartwright RA, Glashan RW, Rogers HJ. The role of N-acetyltransferase in bladder carcinogenesis: a pharmacogenetic epidemiological approach to bladder cancer. Lancet 1982; 2:842–845

7. Tsai YC, Nichols PW, Hiti AL. Allelic losses of chromosomes 9, 11 and 17 in human bladder cancer. Cancer Res 1990; 50:44–47

8. Grossman HB, Liebert M, Antelo M, et al. P53 and Rb expression predict progression in T1 bladder cancer. Clin Cancer Res 1998; 4:829–834

9. Haites N, Schofield A. Inherited predisposition to uro-genital cancers. UroOncology 2001; 1(3): 195–201

10. Cordon-Cardo C, Wartinger D, Petrylak D, et al. Altered expression of the retinoblastoma gene product: prognostic indicator in bladder cancer. J Natl Cancer Inst 1992; 84:1251

11. Prout GR Jr, Barton BA, Griffin PP, Friedell GH. Treated natural history of non-invasive grade I transitional cell carcinoma. J Urol 1992; 148:1413–1419

12. Mariani S, Savige J, Buzza M, Dagher H. Haematuria in asymptomatic individuals. Br Med J 2001; 322:942–943

13. Kincaid-Smith P. Thin basement membrane disease. In: Textbook of nephrology, Massry SG, Glassock RJ (eds). Philadelphia: Lippincott, Williams and Wilkins, 1995; 13:760–764

14. Greene LF, Hanash KA, Farrow GM. Benign papilloma or papillary carcinoma of the bladder? J Urol 1973; 110:205–207

15. Epstein JI, Amin MB, Reuter VR, Mostofi FK. The World Health Organization/International Society of Urological Pathology consensus classification of urothelial (transitional cell) neoplasms of the urinary bladder. Am J Surg Pathol 1998; 22:1435–1448

16. Neal AS, Sharples L, Smith K, et al. The epidermal growth factor receptor and the prognosis of bladder cancer. Cancer 1990; 65:1619–1625

17. Sarkis AS, Dalbagni G, Cordon-Cardo C, et al. Nuclear over-expression of p53 protein in transitional cell bladder carcinoma: a marker for disease progression. J Natl Cancer Inst 1993; 85:53–59

18. Sato K, Moriyama M, Mori S. An immunohistologic evaluation of c-erbB-2 gene product in patients with urinary bladder carcinoma. Cancer 1992; 70:2493–2498

19. Cordon-Cardo C, Wartinger D, Petrylak D, et al. Altered expression of the retinoblastoma gene product: prognostic indicator in bladder cancer. J Natl Cancer Inst 1992; 84:1251–1256

20. Fradet Y, Lacombe L. Can biological markers predict recurrence and progression of superficial bladder cancer? Curr Opin Urol 2000; 10:441–445

21. Mohammed SI, Knapp DW, Bostwick DG, et al. Expression of cyclo-oxygenase-2 (COX-2) in human invasive transitional cell carcinoma (TCC) of the urinary bladder. Cancer Res 1999; 59:5647–5650

22. Michaud DS, Spiegelman D, Clinton SK, et al. Fluid intake and the risk of bladder cancer in men. N Engl J Med 1999; 340:1390–1397

23. Zein TA, Milad MF. Urine cytology in bladder tumours. Int Surg 1991; 76:52–54

24. Haleblian GE, Skinner EC, Dickinson MG, Lieskovsky G, Boyd SD, Skinner DG. Hydronephrosis as a prognostic indicator in bladder cancer patients. J Urol 1998; 160: 2011–2014

25. Mansson W. Muscle invasive bladder cancer – clinical presentation, diagnostic work-up and classification. Erice: Italy International School of Urology and Nephrology, 2000

26. Barentsz JO, Witjes JA. Magnetic resonance imaging of urinary bladder cancer. Curr Opin Urol 1998, 8:95–103

27. Jager GJ, Barentsz JO, Oosterhof GO, Witjes JA, Ruijs JHJ. Pelvic adenopathy in prostatic and urinary bladder carcinoma: MR imaging with a three-dimensional T1-weighted magnetization-prepared-rapid gradient-echo sequence. AJR 1996; 167:1503–1507

28. Barentsz JO, Jager GJ, van Vierzen PBJ, et al. Staging urinary bladder cancer after trans-urethral biopsy: the value of fast dynamic

contrast-enhanced MR imaging. Radiology 1996, 201:185–193

29. Letocha H, Ahlstrom H, Malmstrom P-U, Westlin JE, Fasth KJ, Nilsson S. Positron emission tomography with L-methyl-11-C-methionine in the monitoring of therapy response in muscle-invasive transitional cell carcinoma of the urinary bladder. Br J Urol 1994; 74:767–774

30. Bishop MC. The danger of a long urological waiting list. Br J Urol 1990; 65:433–440

31. Mommsen S, Aagaard J, Sell A. Presenting symptoms, treatment delay and survival in bladder cancer. Scand J Urol Nephrol 1983; 17:164–167

32. Gulliford MC, Petruckevitch A, Burney PGJ. Survival with bladder cancer, evaluation of delay in treatment, type of surgeon and modality of treatment. BMJ 1991; 303:437–440

33. Britton JP. Effectiveness of haematuria clinics. Br J Urol 1993; 71:247–252

34. Sells H, Cox R. Undiagnosed macroscopic haematuria revisited: a follow-up of 146 patients. BJU Int 2001; 88:6–8.

35. Kouriefs C, Leris AC, Mokbel K, Carpenter R. The role of urine cytology in the assessment of lower urinary tract symptoms. BJU Int 2000; 83:1155.

36. Hasan ST, German K, Derry CD. Same day diagnostic service for new cases of haematuria – a district general hospital experience. Br J Urol 1994; 73:152–154

37. Sarosdy MF, deVere White RW, Soloway MS, et al. Results of a multicentre trial using the BTA test to monitor for and diagnose recurrent bladder cancer. J Urol 1995; 154:379–384

38. Utz DC, Farrow GM. Management of carcinoma in situ of the bladder: the case for surgical management. Urol Clin North Am 1987; 533

39. Quilty PM, Duncan V. Treatment of superficial (T1) tumours of the bladder, by radical radiotherapy. Br J Urol 1986; 58:147–152

40. Reading JU, Hall RR, Parmar MKB. The application of a prognostic factor analysis for Ta, T1 bladder cancer in routine urological practice. Br J Urol 1995; 75:604–607

41. Dalesio O, Schulman CC, Sylvester R, de Pauw M, Robinson M, Denis L, members of the EORTC Group. Prognostic factors in superficial bladder tumours: a study of the European Organization for Research on Treatment of Cancer. J Urol 1983; 129:730–733

42. Heney MM, Ahmad S, Flanagan MJ, et al. Superficial bladder cancer: progression and recurrence. J Urol 1983; 130:1083–1086

43. Morales A, Eidinger D, Bruce AW. Intracavitary bacillus Calmette-Guérin in the treatment of superficial bladder tumours. Urology 1976; 116:180–183

44. Oosterlinck W, Kurth KN, Schroeder F, Burtinck J, Hammond B, Sylvester R. A prospective EORTC group randomised trial comparing transurethral resection followed by a single intravesical instillation of epirubicin or water in single stage Ta, T1 papillary carcinoma of the bladder. J Urol 1993; 149:749–752

45. Soloway MS. Rationale for intensive intravesical chemotherapy for superficial bladder cancer. J Urol 1980; 123:461–466

46. Tolley DA, Parmar MKB, Grigor KM, Lallemand G, and the Medical Research Council Superficial Bladder Cancer Working Party. The effect of intravesical mitomycin C on recurrence of newly diagnosed superficial bladder cancer: a further report with 7 years of follow up. J Urol 1996; 155:1233–1238

47. Vegt PDJ, Witjes WPJ, Doesberg WN, Debruyne FMJ. A randomized study of intravesical mitomycin C, bacillus Calmette-Guérin, Tice and bacillus Calmette-Guérin RIVM treatment in pTa-pT1 papillary carcinoma and carcinoma in situ of the bladder. J Urol 1995; 153:929–933

48. Vicente J, Laguna MP, Duarte D, Algaba F, Chechille G. Carcinoma in situ as a prognostic factor for G3 pT1 bladder tumours. Br J Urol 1991; 68:380–382

49. Quilty PM, Duncan W, Chisholm GD. Results of surgery following radical radiotherapy for invasive bladder cancer. Br J Urol 1986 ; 58:396–405

50. Dunst J, Sauer R, Schrott KM, et al. Organ-sparing treatment of advanced bladder cancer: a 10 year experience. Int J Radiat Oncol Biol Phys 1994; 30:261–266

51. Shippley WU, Winter KA, Kaufman DS, et al. Phase III trial of neo-adjuvant chemotherapy in patients with invasive bladder cancer, treated with selective bladder preservation, by combined radiation therapy and chemotherapy: initial results of Radiation Therapy Oncology Group 89-03. J Clin Oncol 1998; 16:3576–3583

52. Donat SM, Grimaldi G, McGuire MS. Prostate-invasive bladder carcinoma: accuracy of transurethral biopsy, patterns of disease recurrence, and clinical impact. J Urol 1998; 159(suppl):164

53. Mootha RK, Muezzinoglu B, Kattan MW, Wheeler TM, Lerner SP. Transitional cell carcinoma of the prostate in radical cystectomy specimens. J Urol 1997; 157(suppl):382

54. Sakamoto N, Tsuneyoshi M, Naito S, Kumazawa J. An adequate sampling of the prostate to identify prostatic involvement by urothelial carcinoma in the bladder cancer patients. J Urol 1993; 149:318–321

55. Hardeman SW, Soloway MS. Urethral recurrence following radical cystectomy. J Urol 1990; 144:666–669

56. Freeman JA, Tarter TA, Esrig D, et al. Urethral recurrence in patients with orthotopic ileal neobladders. J Urol 1996; 156:1615–1619

57. Davidson T. Urinary diversion of bladder substitution in patients with bladder cancer. Urol Oncol 2000; 5:224–231

58. Bricker EM. Bladder substitution after pelvic evisceration. Surg Clin N Am 1950; 30:1511–1512

59. Kock NG, Ghoneim MA, Lycke KG, Mahran MR. Urinary diversion to the augmented and valved rectum: preliminary results with a novel surgical procedure. J Urol 1988; 140:1375–1379

60. Fisch M, Wammack R, Hohenfellner R. The sigma-rectum pouch (MAINZ pouch II). In: Continent urinary diversion, Hohenfellner R, Wammack R (eds). Edinburgh: Churchill Livingstone, 1992:163–182

61. Wenderoth UK, Bachor R, Egghart G, et al. The ileal neobladder: experience and results of more than 100 consecutive cases. J Urol 1990; 143: 492–497

62. Rowland RG. Present experience with the Indiana pouch. World J Urol 1996; 14:92–98

63. Woodhouse CR, MacNeily AE. The Mitrofanoff principle: expanding upon a versatile technique. Br J Urol 1994; 74:447–453

64. Abol-Enein H, Ghoneim MA. Serous lined extramural ileal valve: a new continent urinary outlet. J Urol 1999; 161:786–791

65. Stein R, Fichtner J, Thuroff JW. Urinary diversion and reconstruction. Curr Opin Urol 2000; 10: 391–395

66. Mansson A, Mansson W. When the bladder is gone: quality of life following different types of urinary diversion. World J Urol 1999; 17:211–218

67. Hall RR, Charlton MM, Ongena P. Talking with patients about bladder cancer. In: Clinical management of bladder cancer, Hall RR (ed.). London: Arnold, 1999:365–378

68. Akaza H. Advances in chemotherapy of invasive bladder cancer. Curr Opin Urol 2000; 10:453–457

69. Sylvester R, Sternberg C. The role of adjuvant combination chemotherapy after cystectomy in locally advanced bladder cancer: What we do not know and why. Oncology 2000; 11:851–856

70. Pavone-Macaluso M, Sternberg C. Second-line chemotherapy in advanced bladder cancer. Urol Int 2000; 64:61–69

71. Sternberg CN, Yagoda A, Scher HI, et al. M-VAC (methotrexate, vinblastine, doxorubicin and cisplatin) for advanced transitional cell carcinoma of the urothelium. J Urol 1988; 139:461–464

FURTHER READING

General

Droller M. Clinical presentation, investigation and staging of bladder cancer. In: Principles and practice of genitourinary oncology, Raghavan D, Scher HI, Leibel SA, Lange PH (eds). Philadelphia: Lippincott-Raven, 1997

Herr HW, Lam DL, Denis L. Management of superficial bladder cancer. In: Principles and practice of genitourinary oncology, Raghavan D, Scher HI, Leibel SA, Lange PH (eds). Philadelphia: Lippincott-Raven, 1997

Matzkin H, Soloway MS, Hardeman S. Transitional cell carcinoma of the prostate. J Urol 1991; 146:1207–1212

Oosterlinck W, Lobel B, Jakse G, Malmstrom P-U, Stockle M, Sternberg C. Guidelines on bladder cancer. Arnhem: EAU, 2000

Raghavan D, Shipley WV, Hall RR, Richie JP. In: Principles and practice of genitourinary oncology, Raghavan D, Scher HI, Leibel SA, Lange PH (eds). Philadelphia: Lippincott-Raven, 1997.

Bladder substitution

Hautmann RE, Miller K, Steiner U, Wenderoth U. The ileal neobladder: six years of experience with more than 200 patients. J Urol 1993; 150:40–45

Studer U, Danuser H, Hochreiter W, Springer JP, Turner WH, Zingg EJ. Summary of 10 years' experience with an ileal low-pressure bladder substitute combined with an afferent tubular isoperistaltic segment. World J Urol 1996; 14: 29–39

Wallace DM. Ureteric diversion using a conduit: a simplified technique. Br J Urol 1966; 38:522–527

Haematuria

Mariani AJ, Mariani MC, Maccioni C, et al. The significance of adult haematuria: 1000 haematuria evaluations including a risk benefit and cost effectiveness analysis. J Urol 1989; 141:350–355

Advanced bladder cancer

Duncan W, Quilty PM. The results of a series of 963 patients with transitional cell carcinoma of the urinary bladder primarily treated by radical megavoltage X-ray therapy. Radiother Oncol 1986; 7:299–312

Gospodarowicz MK, Warde P. The role of radiation therapy in the management of transitional cell carcinoma of the bladder. Haematol Oncol Clin North Am 1992; 6:147–168

Herr HW. Conservative management of muscle infiltrating bladder cancer: prospective experience. J Urol 1987; 5:1162–1163

5

Transitional tumours of the urinary tract excluding bladder and urethra

When the patient dies the kidneys may go to the pathologist, but while he lives the urine is ours. It can provide us day by day, month by month, and year by year, with a serial story of the major events going on within the kidney [and in the renal pelvis, by cytology]

Thomas Addis, 1948[1]

GENERAL COMMENTARY

These tumours represent less than 1% of all genitourinary tumours. Most tumours are transitional cell carcinomas (TCCs) and many of the features are similar to bladder cancer. Ninety per cent of pelvic tumours are TCCs and 99% of ureteric tumours are TCCs.[2] It is more common in men by a factor of two or three.[2] The frequency increases with age. It is more common in Caucasians than in blacks.[2]

PRESENTATION

Painless and often gross frank haematuria is the usual method of presentation. Occasionally, the tumour may present as flank pain due to obstruction. This obstruction may be gradual, and the pain may be dull.

Since these tumours are often slow growing, the onset of obstruction can be insidious and slow, and renal function can be destroyed with no symptoms.

CLASSIFICATION OF RENAL PELVIS AND URETER CANCER

The TNM (tumour, node, metastasis) staging system for renal pelvis and ureter cancers is shown in Table 5.1.

PATHOLOGY

Almost all these tumours are TCCs. The lower ureter is more frequently involved than the proximal ureter. Bilateral tumours occur in 2–5% of patients.[3] Between 30 and 75% of patients with upper tract tumours develop bladder tumours at some stage.[3]

Table 5.1 TNM classification of renal pelvis and ureter cancers	
Stage	**Finding**
Ta	Noninvasive papillary
Tis	In situ
T1	Subepithelial connective tissue
T2	Muscularis
T3	Beyond muscularis
T4	Adjacent organs, perinephric fat
N1	Single <2 cm
N2	Single >2–5 cm, multiple <5 cm
N3	>5 cm

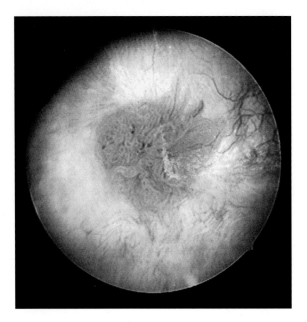

Figure 5.1 Transitional cell cancer protruding from right ureteric orifice.

NATURAL HISTORY

TCC of the urinary tract spreads directly into the kidney or into adjacent structures. High-grade tumours have a greater tendency to spread.

AETIOLOGY

The aetiology is that of bladder tumour (Chapter 4). Stone disease predisposes to squamous cell carcinoma mainly; there is a small increase in incidence in TCC also.[3]

Non-genetic

The aetiological agents are as for bladder cancer. Phenacetin abuse is more common in upper tract tumours.

Families in the Balkans – i.e. Greece, Yugoslavia, Rumania and Bulgaria – may develop an interstitial nephropathy which is known as Balkan nephropathy. The cause is obscure. These people have an increased risk of developing upper urinary tract cancer.[4]

Genetic

Cancer of the ureter and the renal pelvis can be features of hereditary non polyposis colorectal cancer (HNPCC). HNPCC is an autosomal dominant syndrome in which men and women are predisposed to colorectal cancer, but, in addition, women have around a 40% lifetime risk of suffering from endometrial cancer and a 10% lifetime risk of ovarian cancer. Both men and women have additional risks for upper gastrointestinal (GI) tumours and tumours of the ureter and renal pelvis. The condition is associated with mutations in genes involved in DNA mismatch repair.[5]

RISK FACTORS

Risk factors are as for cancer of the bladder, especially smoking. In addition, specifically for upper tract tumours:

- TCC of bladder (3% have upper tract tumours)
- analgesic abuse
- papillary necrosis
- Balkan nephropathy.

DIAGNOSIS

Ultrasound

Ultrasound can show large areas of filling defect in the renal pelvis, or it can show a dilated ureter in lower tract tumours. Only about one-half of investigations are positive.[2]

IVU

Using an intravenous urogram (IVU), a fixed filling defect can be seen in 75–100% of patients.[2]

Cystoscopy

Cystoscopy is mandatory in all such patients since 10% have a concurrent bladder tumour.[2]

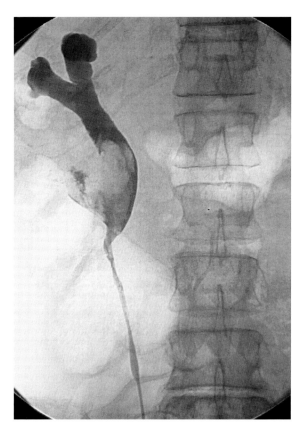

Figure 5.2 Right retrograde pyelogram showing transition cell carcinoma in inferior portion renal pelvis. Note filling defect and under filling of lower pole calyces. The upper pole calyces are distended.

A retrograde pyelogram can be carried out at the same time.

Retrograde pyelogram

Retrograde pyelogram indicates a persistent filling defect which does not move (stones often move slightly). If there is doubt, ultrasound can demonstrate acoustic shadowing, the hallmark of a stone. Seventy-five per cent of patients have a filling defect. There is also a sign called the wine goblet sign that is produced by ureteric dilatation below the filling defect.[2]

Cytology

Cytology has a high false-negative rate for upper tract disease and is positive in only one-third of cases. The yield can be increased using urine from ureteric catheters. Brush biopsies can also be employed.

CT scanning

Computed tomography (CT) can differentiate between a stone and a tumour and aids in staging. It can differentiate between tumour of the kidney and of the renal pelvis. TCCs are usually hypovascular and do not enhance after intravenous contrast.

Ureteroscopy (M309a – diagnostic, M308a – with biopsy)

Ureteroscopy, either with rigid or flexible instruments, allows direct visualisation and biopsy. There is a risk of ureteric perforation occurring in 7% of patients, with the risk of tumour extravasation.

In difficult cases, a percutaneous channel can be made into the renal pelvis and a flexible nephroscope or ureteroscope introduced. There is a theoretical risk of allowing tumour spread in the track and this approach should be used with caution. The pelvis can be irrigated with pure sterile water, but care must be taken to use only small volumes to avoid systemic effects of intravascular haemolysis. A chemotherapy agent such as mitomycin is an alternative.

TREATMENT

Nephro-ureterectomy (OPCS code M0220, M022c) implies removing the entire kidney, ureter and a cuff of bladder. This can be achieved by resecting the ureteric orifice widely and leaving the bladder catheterised for 7 days (M022b). Alternatively, the ureter is traced to the bladder and a cuff of tissue is removed (M022a). A separate incision is required with this approach. A Satinsky clamp can be useful.

Conservative excision

Where the tumour is in the lower portion of the ureter, there is a case for distal ureterectomy and re-implantation. Subsequent follow-up by ureteroscopy is difficult in re-implanted ureters.

Percutaneous treatment (M101a)

Percutaneous extraction of tumour can be employed and this is useful in the very old or where the contralateral kidney has poor function. Follow-up is difficult in these patients and may involve frequent ureteroscopies. There is also a theoretical risk of liberating tumour cells into the access tract.

Ureteroscopic treatment (M278d)

There is a high recurrence rate from local treatment only and there is also a high incidence of ureteric stricture in up to one-third of patients. Very close surveillance is necessary and a balance must be struck between the risk of surgery, the risk of recurrence and the need for repeated general anaesthetics.

Instillation therapy

Mitomycin can be instilled using a nephrostomy but the results, although good, are anecdotal.[3]

Radiation therapy

There are no large trials and, at present, radiotherapy may be used in high-grade disease to achieve local control.

Chemotherapy for advanced disease

A regimen of methotrexate, vinblastine, doxorubicin and cisplatin (M-VAC) has been used with good effect, but there are no randomised controlled trials (RCTs) due to the infrequency of the tumour.

CASE HISTORY (patient permission obtained)

A 79-year-old lady was admitted as an emergency under the care of the physicians, with a 10-day history of frank haematuria. She had been passing bright red urine, with blood clots in it. There was no associated dysuria or dizziness. She had previously been diagnosed as having an arteriovenous malformation (AVM) in her right kidney. However, an abdominal ultrasound revealed a 3 cm solid mass within the upper pole of the left kidney, with mild dilatation of the mid and lower pole calyces of the left kidney. Her right kidney was normal, with no obvious renal masses. The bladder, liver, gallbladder, bile ducts, pancreas and spleen were normal and there was no free fluid seen in the abdomen. A CT scan was arranged.

The CT scan revealed the left kidney to be enlarged and its pelvicalyceal systems grossly distended, with heterogenous material, which on the pre-contrast scan was of high density, consistent with blood. This extended into the proximal left ureter, which was also distended. A few tiny cysts were seen, in addition to small flecks of calcification in the right mid pole and one in the left upper pole of the kidney. There was inflammatory change surrounding the left kidney, which was thought to be the result of pelvicalyceal distension. The left renal cortex enhances to a lesser extent than the right side and there was no contrast excretion into the left pelvicalyceal system. There was duplication of the right renal vein, which probably indicated the site of the previously identified vascular anomaly. There was also a supplementary mesenteric vein, which originated posterior to the sigmoid colon and travelled in a cranial direction anterior to the left psoas muscle, left ureter and left renal vein, to join the splenic vein. Once again, this was thought to be related to the large AVM noted on previous angiography.

The conclusion from the CT scan was that they could not be certain as to whether this was due to an AVM of the left kidney or an underlying pelvicalyceal tumour.

A decision was made to undertake ureteroscopy and this revealed a TCC in her left ureter, G1 pTa.

In view of her age and other medical problems, it was felt that a left nephro-ureterectomy would be the most expeditious way of dealing with her. She was admitted and had the left ureteric orifice resected, using a resectoscope and then the left kidney and ureter were removed en bloc, without the need for a separate incision. She has been followed up since then, with normal chest X-rays, urea and electrolytes and normal check cystoscopies. She is now on annual flexible cystoscopy and has been clear for 3 years.

Comment

In a younger patient, this might have been suitable for a limited resection, but in view of the patient's age and the AVM, it was deemed wiser to carry out a left nephro-ureterectomy, which has, in her case, worked well.

TRANSITIONAL CELL TUMOUR OF THE PROSTATE

General commentary

This is a rare tumour of the prostate. It is usually found after biopsy or at TURP (transurethral resection of prostate). Most cases represent metastatic spread or reimplantation of coexisting bladder tumours. It is, of course, exclusively found in men. It usually presents with haematuria, although irritative symptoms of the prostate, such as frequency, may be discerned by the patient.

Classification

Classification is divided into those who have involvement on the surface and those who have involvement in the prostatic ducts. This can only be determined at histological examination (Table 5.2).

Table 5.2 Summary of classification of transitional cell carcinoma of prostate (prostatic urethra)

Stage	Finding
Tis pu	In situ, prostatic urethra
Tis pd	In situ, prostatic ducts
T1	Subepithelial connective tissue
T2	Prostatic stroma, corpus spongiosum, periurethral muscle
T3	Corpus cavernosum, beyond prostatic capsule, bladder neck (extraprostatic extension)
T4	Other adjacent organs (bladder)

Pathology

The pathology is that of a TCC.

Natural history

If TCC of the prostate is left untreated, this almost inevitably leads to metastases, although the patient's survival may be dictated by the prognosis of the almost invariable coexistent bladder tumour.

Aetiology

The aetiology is that of a bladder tumour.

Non-genetic
As for bladder cancer.

Risk factors

As for bladder cancer.

Previous surgery
Resection of bladder tumour is almost invariable.

Diagnosis

Diagnosis is made by cystoscopy and biopsy or TURP.

Treatment

Because of the small numbers of this type of tumour, there is no guidance from RCTs. Treatment should be based on the patient's age.

BCG (bacille Calmette-Guérin) instillations can occasionally be helpful and may be combined with TURP.

In a young patient with aggressive disease, without metastases, there is an argument for cystoprostatectomy.

Mitomycin has occasionally been used also, but the difficulty in treating the prostate with any intravesical agent is the short dwell time that the drug has in contact with the prostatic epithelium.

REFERENCES

1. Addis T. Glomerular nephritis: diagnosis and treatment. New York: Macmillan, 1948
2. Brooks JD, Marshall FF. Transitional cell carcinoma of the upper urinary tract. In: Principles and practice of genitourinary oncology, Raghavan D, Scher HI, Leibel SA, Lange P (eds). Philadelphia: Lippincott-Raven, 1996
3. Messing EM, Catalona W. Urothelial tumours of the urinary tract. In: Campbell's urology, 7th edn, Walsh PC, Retik AB, Vaughan E, Wein AJ (eds). Philadelphia: WB Saunders, 1997
4. Markovic B. Endemic nephritis and urinary tract cancer in Yugoslavia, Bulgaria and Rumania. J Urol 1972; 107:212
5. Haites N, Schofield A. Inherited predisposition to uro-genital cancers. UroOncology 2000; 1(3): 195–201

FURTHER READING

Epstein JI, Amin MB, Reuter VR, Mostoff FK. The World Health Organization/International Society of Urological Pathology Consensus Classification of Urothelial (Transitional Cell) Neoplasms of the Urinary Bladder. Am J Surg Pathol 1998; 22: 1435–1448

Matzkin H, Soloway MS, Hardeman S. Transitional cell carcinoma of the prostate. J Urol 1991; 146: 1207–1212

Sternberg CN, Yagoda A, Scher HI, et al. M-VAC (methotrexate, vinblastine, doxorubicin and cisplatin) for advanced transitional cell carcinoma of the urothelium. J Urol 1988; 139:461–469

Vicente J, Laguna MP, Duarte D, Algaba F, Chechille G. Carcinoma in situ as a prognostic factor for G3 pT1 bladder tumours. Br J Urol 1991; 68: 380–382

6

Kidney cancer: RCC, variants and Wilms' tumour

The kidneys are of a glandular nature, but redder in colour, like the liver, rather than like the mammae and testicles; for they too, too, are glands but of a whiter colour . . . their cavities are small and like sieves, for the percolation of the urine; and these have attached to each of them nervous canals like reeds, which are inserted into the shoulders of the bladder on each side.

Aretaeus the Cappadocian (AD 81–138)[1]

Servari non potest cui renes vulnerati sunt
(You cannot save a patient whose kidneys are damaged – now fortunately not the case!)

Celsus (25 BC–AD 50)[2]

GENERAL COMMENTARY

The most common (85%) malignant tumour of the kidney in adults is the renal cell carcinoma (RCC), which comprise 3% of all adult malignancies. An estimated 95,000 deaths occur worldwide from this cause per year.[3] About 25% of patients present with metastases.

RCC has been given various terms in the past: the term hypernephroma has been used. This term is both inaccurate and misleading and is mentioned, only to be condemned.

Changes in imaging, with increased use of ultrasound and computed tomography (CT) scanning are identifying more tumours at an earlier stage, with between 20 and 40% being found incidentally.

Renal masses may be benign or malignant.

Benign renal tumours

These give rise to diagnostic confusion.

Angiomyolipomata

There are numerous other types of renal tumours, many of which are benign, such as renal angiomyolipoma, which may occur on its own, or as part of a syndrome known as tuberous sclerosis. This is an autosomal dominant condition associated with mental deficiency and red angiofibromatous papules seen on the face, thickened plaques on the trunk (shagreen patches) and periungual fibromas (smooth nodules beside the nails). The tumours may be bilateral and are noted for their unusual blood vessels, clusters of fat cells and sheets of smooth muscle. The presence of fat in these tumours is almost pathognomonic of an angiomyolipoma. They are often seen incidentally in patients who have CT scans for other reasons. They have negative Hounsfield Units (HU; attenuation units) which indicate fat. About 10% require exploration to make a definitive diagnosis.

Large tumours may cause local discomfort. They may be slow growing and can be removed in part surgically. However, it is perfectly reasonable to leave them alone, assuming the patient does not have symptoms. Embolisation has been an effective treatment in dealing with them. Any surgical operation should be essentially conservative.

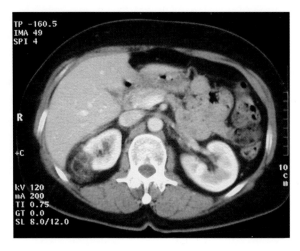

Figure 6.1 CT image of angiomyolipoma of right kidney. Note mixed fat and soft tissue attenuation.

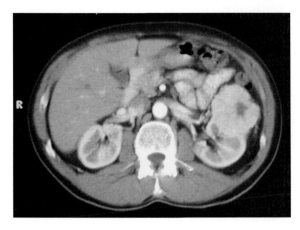

Figure 6.2 CT image of oncocytoma arising in left kidney. Note central stellate non-enhancing appearance (arrow).

Oncocytoma

The other main neoplasm which occurs in the kidney is that of the renal oncocytoma, which usually pursues a benign course. Pathologically it is said to have large cells, with a granular cytoplasm and a rather typical polygonal shape. Mitoses are rare. As long as these features may be seen in renal tumours, one of the features which assists the pathologist in making the distinction is the degree of differentiation.

Renal oncocytomas have a typically quite brown colour, a well-delineated pseudocapsule. They tend to have a central scar, which is noted on the CT or magnetic resonance imaging (MR) scan and often allow the diagnosis to be made preoperatively. They may reach a large size and are usually solitary, but 6% may be bilateral. Usually, they are discovered incidentally,[4] but may give rise to haematuria.

They are only mentioned because of the difficulty in differential diagnosis. A small proportion has been said to metastasise and, where this has happened, the initial diagnosis must be in considerable doubt.[5]

Renal cysts

Renal cysts are often detected on ultrasound. They have a round appearance and a thin wall. Any internal echoes on ultrasound give rise to concern regarding a benign diagnosis.

Bosniak[6] described four categories:

1. Cysts which have a low density of less than 20 HU on CT and do not enhance with intravenous contrast. These are simple cysts without any doubt or malignant potential.
2. Complex cysts which have thin smooth septa. They are minimally complex on CT. Smooth plaques of fine linear calcification can be seen in the wall. High-density cysts of 10–100 HU from previous haemorrhage are included in this category. On MR, blood in a cyst gives a high T1- and T2-weighted image.
3. These cysts have thick septa and may have nodules on the wall and irregular calcification of the wall or septa. These have a moderate probability of malignancy and require surgical evaluation.
4. Although these lesions are cystic, they carry an overwhelming probability of being malignant.

Aspiration under ultrasound control yields fluid which can be sent for cytology. The presence of blood in the aspirate gives some cause for concern. Aspiration also identifies an abscess or an infected cyst.

RENAL CELL CARCINOMA

Epidemiology

This is a relatively rare tumour, contributing 3% to adult malignancies. It is twice as common in males than females (2:1). The incidence of disease appears to be static, but newer forms of imaging and the widespread use of ultrasound are detecting tumours at an earlier stage.[7]

Incidence

The incidence of cancer of the kidney is shown in Table 6.1.

Age

Cancer of the kidney occurs in patients mainly in their 40s–60s.[7] International comparison of survival rates from renal cancer (ICD-9 189) for males and females are shown in Tables 6.2 and 6.3, respectively.

Origin

Renal cell carcinomas arise from the proximal convoluted tubule.

Aetiology

Renal cell carcinoma has been reported in families. It is a feature of von Hippel–Lindau (VHL) disease.[10]

It is also seen more commonly in adults with polycystic renal disease, horseshoe kidneys and acquired renal cystic disease from uraemia.

Trichlorethylene exposure, used in the dry cleaning industry, has been reported to increase incidence.[11] There is a slight association with cigarette smoking, high protein diets, diuretic use, essential hypertension, high red meat intake and obesity. Exposure to cadmium may predispose to development of RCC.[12]

Genes

Cytogenetics shows the most consistent chromosomal changes are deletions and translocations, that involve the short arm of chromosome 3 (3p).

About 1% of all cases are familial: this 1%, however, is important, as predisposition in these families may result in avoidable deaths and morbidity. The familial form is characterised by:

- an early age of onset compared to sporadic cases
- frequent bilaterality
- multicentricity
- mean age at diagnosis in familial cases is 45 years compared to 60 years for sporadic cases.

Renal cell carcinoma is a major feature in several syndromes, including von Hippel–Lindau disease, tuberous sclerosis and a rare familial form in which there is a chromosomal translocation involving chromosome 3p and 8q. In addition, a dominant form of papillary renal cell carcinoma exists.

Von Hippel–Lindau disease (VHL)

Von Hippel–Lindau disease is an autosomal dominant condition with a birth incidence of approximately 1 in 35,000.[10] The most frequent manifestations of this condition are retinal angioma (60%), cerebellar angioma (60%), spinal (13–44%) and brainstem haemangioblastoma (18%), renal cell carcinoma (28%) and phaeochromocytoma (7–20%). In addition, renal, pancreatic and epididymal cysts are frequent findings.

VHL has a penetrance which is age-dependent (0.19 by 15 years, 0.52 by 25 years and 0.91

Table 6.1 Age-standardised incidence rates and standard errors (SE) per 100,000 for cancer of kidney (ICD-9: 189)[8]

Country	Male	±SE	Female	±SE
Zimbabwe, Harare: African	1.7	0.58	0.7	0.26
Zimbabwe, Harare: European	2.9	1.66	2.7	1.69
Argentina, Concordia	3.2	1.13	3.3	1.00
Brazil, Goiania	3.2	0.59	2.6	0.45
Ecuador, Quito	2.6	0.41	1.3	0.26
Peru, Lima	3.4	0.30	2.0	0.21
US, Puerto Rico	4.0	0.24	2.4	0.17
Uruguay, Montevideo	10.6	0.67	3.8	0.35
Canada	11.1	0.12	5.9	0.08
US, SEER:[a] White	10.8	0.14	5.5	0.10
US, SEER: Black	11.8	0.49	5.9	0.30
China, Shanghai	2.9	0.12	1.6	0.09
Hong Kong	3.8	0.16	2.3	0.12
India, Bombay	2.0	0.13	0.9	0.09
Israel: all Jews	10.4	0.32	5.4	0.22
Israel: non-Jews	3.3	0.60	1.8	0.40
Japan, Hiroshima	7.8	0.52	3.2	0.3
Korea, Kangwa	1.8	0.81	1.2	0.63
Kuwait: non-Kuwaitis	4.9	1.44	3.3	1.08
Kuwait: Kuwaitis	2.1	0.61	1.9	0.63
Philippines, Manila	4.0	0.30	2.6	0.21
Singapore: Chinese	4.3	0.32	2.2	0.22
Vietnam: Hanoi	0.6	0.16	0.4	0.11
Austria, Tyrol	14.6	0.92	7.3	0.59
Czech Republic	16.9	0.24	8.5	0.15
Denmark	8.9	0.22	5.7	0.18
Finland	12.1	0.26	6.7	0.18
France, Calvados	8.1	0.69	3.6	0.42
Germany: Eastern States	13.8	0.28	6.8	0.17
Germany: Saarland	12.2	0.58	5.6	0.37
Ireland, Southern	6.2	0.64	3.8	0.52
Italy, Genoa	11.0	0.64	5.3	0.54
The Netherlands	10.2	0.17	5.3	0.12
Poland, Warsaw City	13.3	0.59	6.1	0.35
Spain, Zaragoza	6.2	0.46	2.6	0.30
Sweden	10.3	0.18	6.4	0.14
UK, England and Wales	6.9	0.08	3.3	0.06
UK, Scotland	8.1	0.22	4.5	0.16
Yugoslavia, Vojvodina	4.7	0.28	3.0	0.20
South Australia	8.5	0.44	4.8	0.3
US, Hawaii: White	12.1	1.22	3.8	0.68
US, Hawaii: Japanese	7.3	0.83	2.1	0.37
US, Hawaii: Hawaiian	8.6	1.55	3.0	0.86
US, Hawaii: Filipino	4.4	0.96	1.70	0.59
US, Hawaii: Chinese	5.7	1.55	1.5	0.68

[a]SEER = Surveillance, Epidemiology and End Results programme.

Table 6.2 Relative survival (%) of males at 5 years, all ages, patients diagnosed 1985–89[9]	
Country	**Relative survival (%)**
USA	61.7
France	58.0
Netherlands	56.0
Italy	54.0
Spain	53.0
Germany	50.0
Sweden	49.0
Finland	48.0
England and Wales	38.0
Denmark	36.0
Scotland	35.8

Table 6.3 Relative survival (%) of females at 5 years, all ages, patients diagnosed 1985–89[9]	
Country	**Relative survival (%)**
USA	60.1
France	58.0
Germany	55.0
Italy	55.0
Spain	52.0
Finland	51.0
Netherlands	47.0
Sweden	47.0
England and Wales	35.0
Scotland	33.1
Denmark	33.0

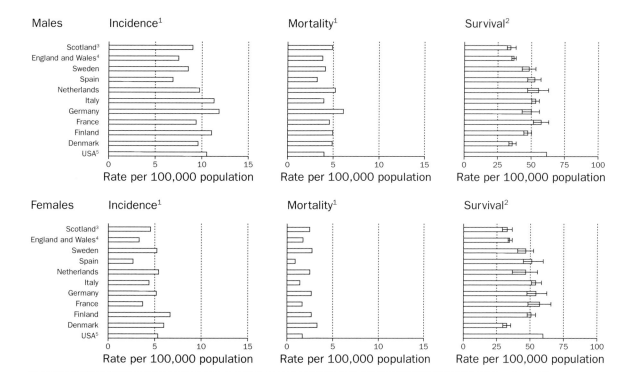

1 Age-standardised rates per 100,000 person-years at risk (World standard population) 1995.
2 Relative survival at 5 years, patients diagnosed 1985–89.
3 Scotland: survival, ages 15–99.
4 England and Wales: incidence 1993; mortality 1995; survival 1986–90 (ages 15–99).
5 USA (SEER, whites): incidence and mortality 1992–96; survival 1989–95.

Figure 6.3 International comparison of incidence, mortality and survival (with 95% CI) of renal cell carcinoma.

by 45 years). By 60 years of age, the risk of cerebellar haemangioblastoma is 84%, of retinal angiomas 70% and of renal cell carcinoma 69%. Since many of these appear at a young age, management criteria have been produced.

Diagnostic criteria for VHL22 [13]
1. For isolated cases, two or more haemangioblastomas (retinal or central nervous system (CNS)) or a single haemangioblastoma with a visceral manifestation.
2. If there is a family history of retinal or CNS haemangioblastoma, only one haemangioblastoma or visceral complication is required.
3. Mutation in the VHL gene.

Screening protocols for VHL
For a known affected patient:

1. annual physical examination and urine testing
2. annual direct and indirect ophthalmoscopy
3. MR (or CT) brain scan every 3 years to age 50 and every 5 years thereafter
4. annual abdominal MRI or ultrasound scan (CT scan every 3 years if followed by ultrasound, or more frequently if multiple renal cysts present)
5. annual 24-hour urine collection for catecholamines and vanillylmandelic acids (VMAs)

For an at-risk relative:

1. annual physical examination, including blood pressure and urine testing
2. annual direct and indirect ophthalmoscopy from age 5 until 60
3. MR (or CT) brain scan every 3 years from 15 to 40 years, and then every 5 years until age 60
4. annual renal MR or ultrasound from age 16 to 65 years
5. annual 24-hour urine collection for catecholamines and VMAs

Management options for VHL [13]
Management is focused on routine surveillance of at-risk individuals, including children, for early detection and treatment of tumours and therapy of known tumours. Use of DNA-based testing for early identification of at-risk family members improves diagnostic certainty and reduces the need for costly screening procedures in those at-risk family members who have not inherited the disease-causing mutation

Multi-drug resistance

Renal cell carcinomas do not normally respond to chemotherapy and this is believed to be due to transmembrane glycoprotein (P170). The MDR1 gene encodes this and this seems to push drugs out of cells more effectively where the gene is present. Multi-drug resistance is not limited to naturally occurring cytotoxics such as vinca alkaloids, anthracyclines and taxanes which are substrates for the glycoprotein membrane efflux pump. Thus, classical multi-drug resistance cannot explain the resistance of renal cancers to drugs such as alkylating agents and platinum complexes, the mechanism of which is currently obscure.

Pathology

Renal cell carcinomas vary in size and can be extremely large. The author has successfully removed one weighing many kilograms, the

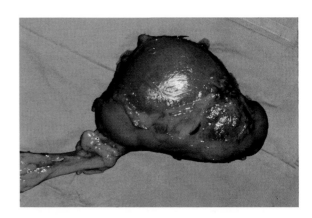

Figure 6.4   Renal cell cancer. Operative specimen.

size of a rugby football. Two per cent of renal tumours are bilateral and often associated with von Hippel–Lindau disease.

The most common pathological diagnosis is that of a clear cell. Granular cell, tubulopapillary and sarcomatoid cells are also identified. Of the 80% which are clear cell, the appearance of the cells is of sheets of cells which are rounded or polygonal, with abundant cytoplasm. They contain lipids and glycogen. Because these are removed in the preparation process, they give rise to this typical appearance.

Variants

Papillary cell carcinoma

Papillary cell carcinoma represents 10% of cases. This is an autosomal dominant condition localised to chromosome 7 – the MET gene. This gene is an oncogene. It is frequently associated with renal dialysis patients with acquired cystic disease. It tends to have a slightly better prognosis than RCC. The cell of origin is also from the proximal convoluted tubule.[14]

Chromophobe cell carcinoma

The cell of origin is from the distal convoluted tubule. The 3p chromosome is absent and although it is keratin positive, it is negative for vimentin. Electron microscopy reveals multiple microvesicles which are said to be diagnostic. It also carries a better prognosis than RCC.

Another rarer variant is the collecting duct carcinoma.[15]

Tumours may contain a variety of different patterns, with clear cell usually predominating. Granular cells, with an eosinophilic cytoplasm, can also be seen.[16]

Fifty per cent of RCCs express a vimentin, and the more vimentin that is seen, the higher grade the tumour is likely to be.

The DNA content of RCCs appears to be prognostic.[17]

Grading

Different grading systems have been proposed. The system proposed by Fuhrman (Table 6.4) has received wide favour and has been shown to relate to survival.

Classification of kidney cancer stage

The TNM (tumour, node, metastasis) staging system for kidney cancers is shown in Table 6.5.

Table 6.4 Fuhrman nuclear grading of renal cell carcinoma[18]

Grade	Characteristics	Occurrence	5-year survival
1	Round, uniform nuclei approximately 10 μm in diameter with minute or absent nucleoli	10%	86%
2	Slightly irregular nuclear contours and diameters of approximately 15 μm with nucleoli visible at 400×	35%	85–25%
3	Moderately to markedly irregular nuclear contours and diameters of approximately 20 μm with large nucleoli visible at 100×	35%	85–25%
4	Nuclei similar to those of grade 3, but also multilobular or multiple nuclei or bizarre nuclei and heavy clumps or chromatin	20%	24%

Table 6.5	TNM classification of kidney cancer
Stage	**Finding**
T1	<7.0 cm; limited to the kidney
T2	>7.0 cm; limited to the kidney
T3	Into major veins; adrenal or perinephric invasion
T4	Invades beyond Gerota's fascia
N1	Single
N2	More than one

Clinical presentation

The classical triad of presentation comprised pain, haematuria and flank mass. Fortunately, this is now much rarer and the majority of patients would normally present with haematuria.

In the past, the patient might have had pain from the size of the tumour, but any pain is now more likely to be due to colic passing clots.

It is imperative that patients with frank haematuria have their upper tracts imaged.

Many renal tumours produce a wide variety of hormones and proteins and almost every protein seems to have been described at some point.

> **Key point:** Rapid evaluation of renal masses is mandatory, since reduction in delay of treatment may improve survival.

Mechanisms of hypertension

Associated with renal cell carcinoma are:[19,20]

- hyperreninaemia
- arteriovenous fistula
- polycythaemia
- hypercalcaemia
- ureteral obstruction
- cerebral metastasis
- Goldblatt effect.

The normal kidney has endocrine functions and, as would be expected, the tumour can occasionally pirate these functions. Because of these curious substances which are elaborated, the patient may present with weight loss, fever, hypertension or hypercalcaemia.

Occasionally, the patient may present with Stauffer syndrome, which is a non-metastatic hepatic dysfunction characterised by abnormal liver function tests, white blood cell abnormality, fever, areas of hepatic necrosis, without hepatic metastases. Removal of the tumour usually rectifies these abnormalities.

Hypercalcaemia has been reported in up to 10% of patients with renal carcinomas. This is usually due to a calcitonin-related protein.

Mechanisms implicated in hypercalcaemia

Associated with renal cell carcinoma with no osseous metastasis are the following humoral factors:

- parathyroid hormone (PTH)
- osteoclast-activating factor
- 1,25-dihydroxyvitamin D3 $(1,25(OH)_2D_3)$
- transforming growth factor (TGF) α and β
- colony-stimulating factor.

Primary hyperparathyroidism
If there are secondaries, however, hypercalcaemia may be due to skeletal metastases.

Paraneoplastic syndromes and renal cancer

Nonspecific syndromes
- Anaemia
- Elevated sedimentation rate
- Coagulopathy
- Reversible hepatic dysfunction
- Fever
- Amyloidosis
- Neuropathy.

Specific syndromes
- Hypercalcaemia
- Erythrocytosis
- Hypertension

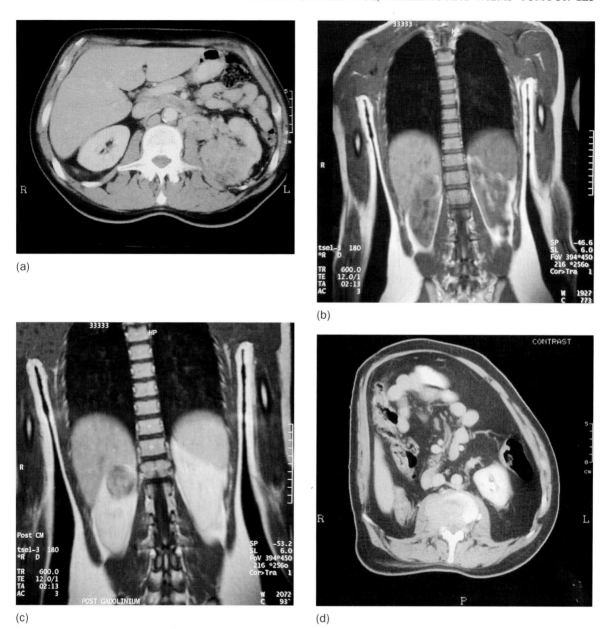

(a)

(b)

(c)

(d)

Figure 6.5 (a) CT image demonstrating left renal carcinoma, invading left renal vein plus enlarged retroperitoneal lymph nodes. (b) Coronal T1 MR primary renal cell carcinoma in upper pole right kidney. (c) Primary renal cell carcinoma in upper pole right kidney showing increased visibility after gadolinium enhancement. (d) CT image of upper abdomen demonstrating vertebral metastasis from renal cell cancer. Note absent right kidney as patient was scanned lying on right side, since pain precluded the customary supine position.

- Elevated human chorionic gonadotrophin (hCG)
- Cushing's syndrome
- Hyperprolactinaemia
- Ectopic insulin/glucagon

High angiotensin levels can cause hypertension, and these can revert to normal after removal of the tumour.

Investigations

Recommended investigations are:

- intravenous urogram (IVU)
- ultrasound
- CT scan
- chest X-ray.

> Renal tumours may not be seen on IVU, particularly if they are small or peripheral.

Ultrasound is able to differentiate a cystic from a solid mass. A cystic mass may have multiple internal echoes. Where there is doubt that the cyst is simple, then a CT scan is mandatory. CT is believed to be the method of choice for staging renal carcinomas. To allow us further staging, an enhanced CT scan allows an estimation of the function of the opposite kidney.

CT is still considered the gold standard for diagnosing renal masses (Figures 6.5a, d).

MR scanning may be less sensitive than CT for solid lesions less than 3 cm in diameter. However, it is able to give good information about invasion of the renal vein and inferior vena cava without requiring a further contrast material.

An MR, with gadolinium can be used in patients who are unable to receive contrast with iodine, e.g. patients with allergy (Figures 6.5b, c). CT angiography (CTA) is replacing conventional diagnostic angiography. It may have a particular role where nephron-sparing surgery is contemplated.[21]

SURGICAL TREATMENT

Radical nephrectomy and excision of perirenal tissue (OPCS code M0210)

Surgery is the most effective means of curing localised renal carcinoma in unilateral and local disease. The surgeon's objective is to remove the kidney en bloc with Gerota's fascia and its contents and the adrenal gland.

Preoperative
- MR scan or
- CT scan
- Blood tests
    haemoglobin
    full blood count
    urea and electrolytes
    liver function tests
- electrocardiography (ECG)
- echocardiography where indicated by significant cardiac disease.

Renography

> It is essential to document the function of the opposite kidney to ensure it has sufficient function.

Cross-matching
A minimum of 4 units of packed cells are cross-matched.

Heparin
It is customary to give the patient 5000 units of heparin subcutaneously twice daily preoperatively and until the patient is ambulant.

Operating theatre allocation
- An operating time of at least 3 hours is booked.
- Two assistants must be free, at least one of whom is experienced.

Consent
This must be obtained preoperatively with the patient non-sedated.

Marking the side

This should be done preoperatively with the patient awake and not sedated

Check the side

Confirm with theatre sister or anaesthetist, i.e. not someone who is junior to you on the same team and who could be overly influenced. Check the side with the X-rays and with reports, preferably using reports that are independent – the radiologist can get it wrong too!

Surgical approach to the kidney

There continues to be debate as to the best approach to the kidney. For large tumours, I prefer an approach through the abdomen. This used to have the added advantage of allowing inspection of the liver, but modern CT scanning makes this argument redundant. It is unlikely that significant metastases have been missed.

The patient is placed on his back. A beanbag is placed under the ribs on the side of the proposed incision. This has the affect of allowing the intestines to move away from the midline to the opposite side.

I prefer a subcostal approach, although a midline one can be satisfactory, but in my experience, requires a longer incision. The preferred incision is from about 1 cm below the xiphisternum, following the lower boundaries of the ribs, through the anterior layer of the rectus sheath, the rectus muscle, extending the incision laterally, through external oblique and internal oblique. This division can be done with cutting diathermy which minimises bleeding, and the sucker can be used to suck smoke. It is helpful if an assistant lifts the anterior abdominal wall, so that there is no unintended damage to the bowel lying beneath.

Once the peritoneal cavity is opened, fingers placed into the cavity ensure no possibility of intestinal damage.

I find it useful to put one large pack in the abdomen, to secure the intestine and then a second pack allows the assistant to control any abdominal contents with his fingers. This allows division of the lateral reflection of the peritoneal cavity off the ascending or descending colon. On the left side, it is important to pay attention to avoid damaging the spleen and constant vigilance is required to avoid this, especially if you have an overenthusiastic assistant.

The ureter is best identified at first opening of the retroperitoneal space. After a small amount of bleeding, the ureter is much more difficult to see. It is worth placing a sloop around the ureter until you are sure that the kidney and tumour can be safely removed. It is much rarer today to be presented with an inoperable tumour, but having divided the ureter prematurely, you are condemning the patient to pain until the kidney ceases to function. What can be worse, is that the ligature can erode and the patient is left with a urinary fistula. The only expedient if the ureter is divided and the kidney cannot be removed safely is to re-anastamose the ureter, prolonging the operation where it could be avoided.

The renal artery should be secured and divided first if possible. Since it lies posterior to the renal vein, it is not always possible and the watchwords should be safety first, and not slavish adherence to surgical dogma. It can occasionally be safer to mobilise a kidney prior to isolating the vessels, since this allows a speedier nephrectomy. Bleeding is much more easily dealt with once the kidney is removed.

Remember that a number of patients will have more than one artery and, quite often, several veins.

Traditionally, the veins were said to be ligated first, but in practice the vessels are usually divided as they present themselves. Once the artery has been ligated, the kidney becoming ischaemic should reassure the surgeon.

The renal vein is divided and, where tumour thrombus is present, an attempt should be made to remove this. This should be known in advance and it is frequently possible to contain any tumour thrombus by isolating the involved segment of vein.

For tumours on the right-hand side, where the renal vein is short, it is possible to place a Satinski clamp over a portion of the inferior vena cava and the tumour may then be easily extracted. A formal vascular closure of the inferior vena cava is of course necessary before releasing the clamp.

Adrenalectomy

There have been a number of trials of whether this is necessary. My approach is if the adrenal is adherent to the specimen, especially if the tumour is upper pole, then it is prudent to take the adrenal. Where the tumour is remote, e.g. lower pole, it is not necessary to remove the adrenal.[22]

Very occasionally, a patient is hypotensive after the removal of the adrenal and requires 100 mg of hydrocortisone intramuscularly.

Hypotension postoperatively is almost always due to blood loss until proved otherwise. Do not be fooled by the absence of blood in a drain – drains block, and clot does not travel through drains easily. A drain may be flushed to increase or test patency, but if the patient is hypotensive with a tachycardia, suspect bleeding.

Lymphadenectomy

There is debate about the role of lymphadenectomy. Where there are a small number of obviously involved nodes, it would be prudent to remove them, but where there are multiple nodes extending up the cava, it is unlikely that extended lymphadenectomy makes much difference, in most cases.

Where a tumour is very large, or where it is upper pole, or where there is suspected involvement of the diaphragm, then a transthoracic approach or thoracoabdominal incision may be used.

Preoperative angiography may be requested, but it has fallen into disfavour. Similarly, preoperative embolisation is occasionally helpful in big vascular tumours, but often merely delays the patient's operation.

Key points
- Prior to nephrectomy, the side of the lesion must be carefully identified and verified by two people, analysing independent reports and checking these with the IVU, CT scan and ultrasound
- Renal function of the contralateral kidney must be ascertained.

There has been no significant benefit seen in preoperative or postoperative radiotherapy.

Laparoscopic radical nephrectomy (OPCS code M0280)

This technique may have a place in special centres. The operation usually takes longer and there may be concern about spilling tumour cells. The advantage is that of earlier discharge from hospital and earlier return to full activity.

Renal sparing (nephron sparing) surgery – partial nephrectomy (M038)

There is increasing interest, particularly with small tumours in conservative operations, preserving the uninvolved portion of kidney. This is suitable for experienced operators in large centres. This is of course particularly applicable if there are bilateral renal tumours.[23,24]

RCC involving the inferior vena cava

In inferior vena cava involvement in a fit patient, where tumour is seen extending far into the inferior vena cava, there is a place for removing the tumour and the thrombus, under cardiac bypass. This can be the case even where the thrombus extends into the right atrium. A 5-year survival of 64% can be achieved.

Locally invasive renal cancer

In large renal cancers, even where there are metastases, it may be judged appropriate to attempt to remove the tumour, because of the painful effects of local invasion of the tumour.

Radiotherapy
These tumours are typically resistant to radiotherapy. The adjacent normal organs (small bowel, stomach, liver, contralateral kidney) limit the dose of radiation which can be safely delivered to the renal bed following nephrectomy for locally advanced disease.

Although postoperative radiotherapy has been given, e.g. where there is tumour extension into Gerota's fascia, there has been no demonstration of benefit in terms of increased survival in these patients.

Embolisation

RCC can be embolised and the procedure can be repeated. This is of use in the elderly or frail. The process is attended by subsequent pain, and it is essentially palliative, being useful for controlling haematuria.

Cryotherapy

There is increasing interest in cryoablation using probes inserted percutaneously, at laparoscopy or at open operation. This is of particular use in bilateral tumours.[25–28]

Radiofrequency ablation

This modality is gaining ground, since the radiofrequency probe can be inserted into the sedated patient using local anaesthetic. Local vessels act as a heat sink, so care is especially needed in central tumours. Peripheral tumours are more easily ablated.

Follow-up after nephrectomy

After successful nephrectomy, the patient will be followed up at an initial postoperative visit and then will be seen at 3 and 6 months. At either or both of these stages, the surgeon may elect to perform imaging of the renal bed, since it is known that local recurrence can be treated surgically and may still be curative.

Subsequent follow-up is based on chest X-rays for 3 years postoperatively. Ultrasound to the renal bed with CT scanning as an alternative should be carried out in advanced local cases, or where nephron sparing surgery has been carried out. Function in the remaining kidney should be assessed by creatinine estimations, or by ultrasound or CT scan if the patient has VHL.

Unfortunately, RCC can return many years later, but, often, surgeons will elect to discharge the patient at around 4 years follow-up.

TREATMENT OF METASTATIC RENAL CANCER

Chemotherapy

Chemotherapy for renal cell cancer has been disappointing. Yagoda and his colleagues reviewed 4093 patients treated with chemotherapy in 83

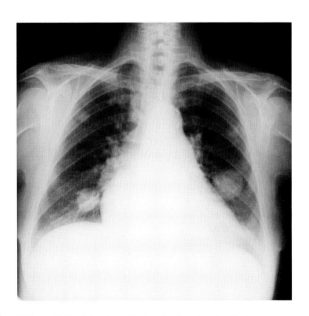

Figure 6.6 Chest radiograph showing typical 'cannonball' metastases from primary renal cell cancer.

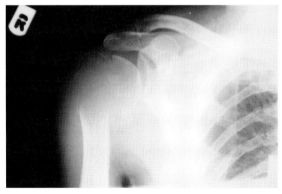

Figure 6.7 Expansive lytic metastasis in right humoral head from primary renal cell carcinoma.

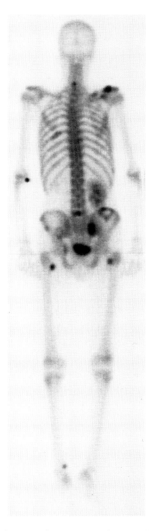

Figure 6.8 Isotope bone scan showing bone metastases from primary renal cell cancer. Note the absent left kidney removed by nephrectomy.

phase II trials and found an overall response rate of 6.8%.[29]

5-Fluorouracil (5-FU) had a response rate of 13.4% and vinblastine, the next best, had a response rate of 6.4%.[30]

Hormonal therapy

Although hormonal treatment enjoyed a vogue in the 1970s, the results are insubstantial, and hormonal treatment is now almost relegated to a palliative measure.

The main hormone employed was medroxy-progesterone acetate (MPA). The response rate to MPA is about 10%.[31]

A 7% response rate with a median survival of 6 months was seen in the recent Medical Research Council (MRC) study comparing MPA to interferon-α.[32]

Tamoxifen, at a dose of 100–150 mg/m² per day, can produce responses of the order of 7%.[30]

> When responses occur to hormones, they can be dramatic and durable, especially where the disease is limited to the lungs.
>
> There appears to be no correlation between response to immunotherapy and response to hormonal therapy.

Immunotherapy

Interferons

Interferons have a wide range of actions:

- antiviral activity
- enhancement of leucocyte-mediated cyto-toxicity
- antiproliferative activity on malignant cells.

Interferon was the first lymphokine to be used clinically. Type 1 interferons are produced by leucocytes and interferon-β is produced by helper T cells. Type 2 interferon (interferon-γ) is produced by T lymphocytes, when stimulated by mitogens.

Interferon-α_2 may be used with some success in treating metastatic disease. Objective responses of 15–20% have been observed.

The MRC study comparing MPA to interferon-α in a dosage of 10 mega units subcutaneously three times a week showed a 14 vs 7% advantage in response and a survival advantage of 8.5 months versus 6 months in favour of interferon-α.[32] The best responses are seen in patients with good prognostic features. Interferon-γ has not shown the same response rates or survival advantage.[33]

There are ongoing trials to find more optimal treatments. The MRC are examining interferon-α versus the Atzpodien regime in metastatic disease in patients with good performance status.

The European Organization for Research and Treatment of Cancer (EORTC) are trialling adjuvant immunotherapy (again, the Atzpodien regime) vs no systemic treatment following nephrectomy for node-positive renal cancer.

Interleukins

Interleukin-2 (IL-2), is a T-cell growth factor, has been shown to produce lymphokine activated killer cells (LAK cells) and enhances the function of LAK cells. Initially, IL-2 was tried in isolation, and then was combined with adoptive cellular therapy, using LAK cells.

Some excellent results were observed in a small number of patients, but the addition of LAK cells did not seem to make significant difference. It would appear that the disease often recurs when the IL-2 therapy is withdrawn. Response rates of 15–20% have been reported.

IL-2 therapy has numerous side effects, such as fever, chills, vomiting and renal and cardiovascular effects.[34]

The Atzpodien regimes

Atzpodien reported response rates of 49% with acceptable toxicity with a combination of bolus 5-FU, subcutaneous interferon-α and IL-2.[35] Overall survival was increased to 42 months.

A number of similar studies have been reported and there has been interest in protracted venous infusion of 5-FU; a wider benefit, even in patients with widespread disease, has been claimed.

Nephrectomy in patients with metastatic RCC

There may be four reasons for nephrectomy in these patients:

- Nephrectomy can palliate, especially where pressure from the tumour is causing symptoms.
- Occasionally (<1%), regression of metastases or involution has been seen, and the author has met clinicians who have had such cases, even where the secondaries have been proven by biopsy.
- In isolated cases where there is a solitary liver or lung secondary, nephrectomy and resection of isolated secondaries can be undertaken. This is only worthwhile in younger fit patients, and is not useful as a general rule.
- Nephrectomy also reduces the bulk of tumour where biological agents are to be used.

It has recently been shown that nephrectomy increases survival by a number of months in the presence of metastases. This option can be offered to patients if their expected survival will allow them to enjoy any increased survival. It is a mistake to inflict an operation on a patient who will be unlikely to leave hospital, and may be in postoperative discomfort until their death.

Factors with predictive value for response to systemic treatment

- Nephrectomy
- Long disease-free interval
- Good performance status
- Absence of visceral metastasis other than lung
- Relatively small tumour burden.

Renal cell prognostic factors

- Single site of metastatic disease
- Stage
- Grade
- Nuclear morphometry
- DNA content
- Cytogenetic findings
- Vascular invasion
- Clinical and laboratory variables
- Weight loss
- Performance status
- Erythropoietin levels.

Renal case history 1 (patient permission obtained)

A 73-year-old retired engine driver originally presented with a history of irritative bladder symptoms, frequency, nocturia and intermittent flow, with some urgency. He had been treated with finasteride, but this had not been of any benefit. He had no past history of any note.

On examination his abdomen was unremarkable. He had a small, clinically benign prostate. A flow rate was attempted at the clinic, but this was an inadequate volume. He was also noted to have a trace of blood and protein on urinalysis.

It was arranged for him to attend for a flexible cystoscopy and ultrasound of his urinary tract. His ultrasound was grossly abnormal and showed bilateral hydronephrosis but, in addition, he had a lobulated solid T1 mass measuring 5 cm × 5 cm × 6 cm in the medial upper pole in the right-hand side. This was felt to be consistent with a renal tumour. There was also a filling defect in his bladder, which was in fact a large bladder stone. There were also some cysts in his liver.

It was arranged for him to attend for a CT scan and a kidney, ureter and bladder (KUB) (the latter because of his bladder stone). Because of the difficulties in reviewing his scan, he was discussed at our X-ray conference. There were in fact four abnormalities noted:

1. a right renal mass, which was almost certainly tumour
2. a lower pole abnormality of the left kidney – aetiology was obscure
3. a bizarre appearance in the bladder, probably due to a bladder stone
4. liver cysts.

It was felt that because the right renal mass was unequivocally tumour T1, arrangements were made for him to attend for a right radical nephrectomy.

At operation, he had an open cystolithotomy, removing several large stones and also excising a bladder diverticulum.

He also had a right radical nephrectomy and he made a good recovery from this. Not sur-prisingly, he failed a trial without catheter and was discharged home with a long-term catheter.

He subsequently underwent an angiogram for his left renal abnormality and it was felt that a partial nephrectomy would be possible, but he was warned that he might lose the entire kidney and it was also felt that he might require dialysis.

He was admitted as an emergency with confusion, dehydration and a urinary tract infection, with associated haematuria. This responded well to intravenous cefotaxime and fluids, and he improved markedly.

He was allowed home and 1 month later we admitted him for re-staging of his left kidney.

There appeared to be no change in the left lower pole tumour – T1. He therefore underwent partial nephrectomy, which was carried out uneventfully. He required a transfusion during surgery, but has been reviewed 6 weeks following his surgery and his haemoglobin is normal at 136 g/l, with a marginally elevated urea of 9.1 mmol/l and a creatinine of 153 mmol/l.

At present he has been placed on finasteride because of his prostate problems and is being reviewed 3 monthly.

Histology
- Right kidney: there was a yellowish tumour 6 cm in diameter at the upper pole. The tumour was composed of cords of clear cells, with a moderate-sized nucleus (average size 15 μm diameter – grade 2). The features are those of a usual clear cell renal carcinoma. The distal ureteric resection margin appeared normal, although the ureter and pelvis showed moderate nonspecific chronic inflammatory cell infiltration in the lamina propria. The renal vessels at the hilum are free from tumour.
- Left kidney: clear cell adenocarcinoma was identified in the left kidney, with central degeneration. Macroscopically, no hilar vessels were seen. The pathologist comments that it was difficult to comment on the adequacy of excision.

Renal case history 2 (patient permission obtained)

A 55-year-old male presented with moderately raised blood pressure, at 130/94. He had ++ of protein and ++ blood in his urine and he had had a history of frequency; a diagnosis of presumed urinary tract infection was made by his general practitioner.

He was started on trimethoprim and urine was sent for culture. No growth was obtained from the culture.

He developed some iliac fossa pain and a slightly tender prostate. His antibiotics were changed to ciprofloxacin and he was feeling much better 1 week later. His urinalysis was negative and his mid-stream specimen of urine (MSSU) showed no growth. His was noted to have a slightly raised alkaline phosphatase, a creatinine of 135 mmol/l and urea of 4.5 mg/dl. His prostate-specific antigen (PSA) was normal at 0.6.

He went for an offshore medical and, because of slight breathlessness on exertion, a chest X-ray was performed. This revealed multiple round opacities in the lung fields, with a little fluid in the right base. The appearances were consistent with secondary deposits, possibly renal in origin.

He was therefore referred urgently to my clinic. At this point he was noted to have persistent haematuria.

On examination he was pale and showed evidence of some weight loss. He had a bulky right loin mass, suggestive of a renal carcinoma. He had a small soft prostate. An ultrasound was obtained and a further chest X-ray. The chest X-ray confirmed the previous findings, with multiple cannonball-type metastases throughout both lung fields.

An abdominal ultrasound confirmed the presence of a large right-sided renal mass, which was contained within the capsule. There was also evidence of a right pleural effusion. The renal vein could not be visualised. In view of the metastatic nature of the disease, he was seen urgently by the medical oncologists. The treatment options were discussed with the patient and his wife.

He was started initially on interferon 5 mega units three times a week, given subcutaneously. Routine bloods were taken for a baseline, as was a further chest X-ray.

He had developed some feelings of nausea and his interferon was reduced to 5 mega units twice weekly.

He required emergency admission following this, because the large right-sided pleural effusion was found to be hypercalcaemic. His interferon was clearly no longer controlling his disease and the treatment was discontinued.

His effusion was drained and his hypercalcaemia corrected with intravenous fluids and pamidronate. His systemic treatment was changed to Megace (megestrol acetate) 160 mg twice a day.

He required admission 1 month later for recurrent malignant hypercalcaemia, which improved with intravenous fluids, pamidronate and a blood transfusion.

The following month he required further treatment with pamidronate. He had an infusion over 2 hours. He was reviewed 1 month later and was doing remarkably well.

At his most recent visit, he is continuing on his Megace and pamidronate. His chest X-ray showed almost complete resolution of the pulmonary metastases.

The long-term outlook must, of course, remain guarded.

NEPHROBLASTOMA – WILMS' TUMOUR

Wilms' tumour occurs in 1 in 200,000 children per year, mainly in the 3rd year; almost all cases occur within the first 5 years of life. This is the second most common abdominal tumour in childhood.

Aetiology

Non-genetic
None recognised.

Genetic
One per cent of cases have been found to have a family history. It is often associated with

congenital abnormalities, such as aniridia, hemihypertrophy and various genitourinary abnormalities known as the WAGR syndrome.

The WAGR syndrome is now known to be a contiguous gene syndrome in which several genes lying next to each other on chromosome 11p13 are deleted.

Most patients with Wilms' tumour and aniridia have a constitutive deletion at 11p13 which is present in all cells of their body at that position. Genes at this locus include WT1 and the aniridia gene PAX6.

Another Wilms' tumour gene, WT2, has been mapped to chromosome 11p15 by loss of heterozygosity studies in tumour specimens.[36]

Pathology of Wilms' tumour

Tumours can arise in any part of the kidney, but the majority are in the upper pole. A pseudocapsule of connective tissue surrounds the tumour.

The tumour may have a lobular appearance, with fibrous septa. There may be cystic degeneration within the tumour. The surrounding renal tissue can be damaged by compression or by infiltration. Poorly formed tubular structures or glomerular structures may be surrounded by primitive mesenchymal cells, which can form recognisable elements, striated muscle, fat or even bone.

Congenital mesoblastic nephroma
There is a variant of the condition called congenital mesoblastic nephroma and surgery alone is curative.

There are subgroups of nephroblastoma, which have sarcomatous or anaplastic histology. It is imperative that an experienced paediatric pathologist examines these tumours, since the precise histology may dictate the best form of treatment.

Clinical presentation

Most cases of nephroblastoma present as an asymptomatic abdominal mass. About one-third of patients have abdominal pain and less than 25% have haematuria. An ultrasound will show distortion of the calyces and this can be confirmed on an IVU. CT scanning has become routine practice.

Staging
The most commonly used staging system is the National Wilms' Tumour Study (Table 6.6).

Treatment
It is important that children with this disease are managed by experienced clinicians to help us to obtain the expected 80% cure rate.

Surgery is normally employed to remove the primary tumour. Occasionally, preoperative chemotherapy and/or radiation may be used prior to surgical treatment.

The kidney is exposed through a transverse abdominal incision and any tumour thrombus must be isolated prior to ligating the renal vein. A standard radical nephrectomy is carried out, along with sampling of any regional lymph nodes. In areas where there is thought to be residual tumour, tissues are marked with clips.

Radiotherapy
Radiotherapy is normally started within 2 weeks of surgery. The fields are used to compass the tumour bed and adjacent lymph nodes.

Table 6.6	Wilms' tumour staging system
Stage	**Finding**
1	Tumour localised to kidney and completely resected
2	Tumour extending beyond the kidney but completely resected
3	Residual tumour confined to abdomen, e.g. gross peritoneal contamination, lymphatic metastases
4	Distant metastases
5	Bilateral involvement

Protection must be given to important growth sites, such as the contralateral ovary in girls, and femoral heads and acetabula should be protected with lead blocks.

Chemotherapy

Chemotherapy regimes are changing, with a combination of vincristine and actinomycin D. Accurate staging is necessary to gauge which children need chemotherapy.

Complications

- Hair loss
- Vincristine neuropathy, which may present as abdominal pain or ileus
- Hepatitis
- Severe thrombocytopenia
- Oedema (especially after hepatic radiation, following a course of actinomycin D at full dosage).

Follow-up

- Monthly for the 1st year
- Two monthly for the 2nd year
- At each follow up chest X-ray (postero-anterior and lateral)
- Dimercaptosuccinic acid (DMSA) scans at 6 and 12 months
- Urea and electrolytes every 6 months
- Blood pressure every 6 months
- MSSUs.

Adult Wilms' tumour – case history

A 23-year-old man had a 2-month history of left loin pain. This became increasingly worse and he was admitted as an emergency. He had previously been well, with no family history of note. He is a single male, living with his uncle. On examination he had no lymphadenopathy and his chest was clear. The liver was not palpable.

An ultrasound on the day of admission showed replacement of his left kidney by tumour and a normal right kidney, liver and spleen. An ultrasound-guided biopsy was unhelpful and a left nephrectomy was undertaken.

At operation there was a large retroperi-toneal mass, but no lymphadenopathy. A large amount of clot was evacuated from around the renal hilum and the renal pedicle was clamped. The kidney and perinephric fat capsule were removed.

At histology, the left nephrectomy specimen measured $14\,cm \times 7\,cm \times 9\,cm$. The kidney was covered by blood clot and the hilar area was irregular. There was an $11\,cm \times 6\,cm$ tumour occupying most of the kidney.

Histologically, the tumour was highly cellu-lar and almost completely nectrotic, with areas of haemorrhage. The surviving renal parenchyma showed interstitial fibrosis, with almost complete atrophy of the tubules, sug-gesting a pre-existing abnormality. A block from the hilum shows widespread infiltration by tumour of essentially blastema type. Focal tubal formation was noted and the tumour cells were positive for cytokeratin. The features were those of a poorly differentiated carcinoma of kidney and the presence of tubular differentia-tion suggested the possibility of a nephroblas-toma (Wilms' tumour), despite the patient's age.

Histology of the renal capsule showed wide-spread haemorrhage and patchy infiltration by necrotic anaplastic carcinoma cells. Tubule for-mation was present within the fibrous tissue of the capsule.

The oncologists saw him, and initial chemotherapy was delayed due to neutropenia. A chest X-ray remained clear and he was started on vincristine and adriamycin (doxoru-bicin hydrochloride).

After finishing his adjuvant chemotherapy, a CT scan showed no evidence of residual tumour from 3 months after his initial surgery. Almost 1 year from his original surgery, a rou-tine chest X-ray showed a left apical mass. A CT scan suggested that this was localised and that there was no evidence of any metastatic disease elsewhere, nor of any local recurrence.

Because this was believed to be a solitary metastasis, the thoracic surgeons saw him. At thoracotomy, this solitary metastasis was removed with a wedge of lung.

Unfortunately, the mediastinal nodes appeared to be involved and these were removed. Histology confirmed a recurrence of his nephroblastoma. He was therefore given radiotherapy. Apart from some mild oesophagitis, he had no other symptoms.

He was followed up closely over a 2-year period and, 25 months after presentation, routine chest X-ray showed a further relapse, with a retrocardiac mass in the left lung, measuring 5 cm in diameter. In addition there was a separate 9 mm lesion in the left upper lobe and mediastinal lymphadenopathy.

He was started on second-line chemotherapy, with etoposide and cisplatin. He experienced no significant toxicities from his first cycle and his performance status remained at 0. He completed four cycles of EP chemotherapy and he then had a successful peripheral stem cell collection. He was then re-admitted for high-dose chemotherapy with carboplatin, etoposide and cyclophosphamide.

He was warned of the symptoms of moderately severe toxicity, with nausea and vomiting, mucositis and diarrhoea and a period of profound myelosuppression until his stem cells engrafted. He had initial problems with his Hickman line. He was started on G-CSF (granulocyte colony-stimulating factor) on day +1.

His neutropenic phase was complicated by fever, requiring broad-spectrum intravenous antibiotics and intravenous amphotericin B. He had a short period of parenteral nutrition. He had a rapid neutrophil engraftment, with neutrophils rising and he was given nebulised pentamidine as chest prophylaxis and was also kept on acyclovir prophylaxis for 3 months.

He was seen some 3 weeks following his transplant reinfusion and was well. The scan showed complete response and he is at present keeping well, although the long-term outlook must remain guarded.

REFERENCES

1. Aretaeus the Cappadocian. On the affections about the kidneys. In: The extant works of Aretaeus the Cappadocian, Adamas F (ed.). Birmingham, Alabama: Classics of Medicine Library, 1990

2. Celsus 25 BC–AD 50. De Medecina, translated by WG Spencer. Birmingham, Alabama: Classics of Medicine Library, 1989

3. Webb A, Gore M. The management of metastatic renal cell cancer. UroOncology 2000; 1:1–6

4. Tsui K, Shvarts O, Smith R, Figlin R, deKernion J, Belldegrun A. Renal cell carcinoma: prognostic significance of incidentally detected tumors. J Urol 2000; 163:426–430

5. Morra M, Das S. Renal oncocytoma: a review of histogenesis, histopathology, diagnosis and treatment. J Urol 1993; 150:295–302

6. Bosniak MA. Problems in the radiologic diagnosis of renal parenchymal tumors. Urol Clin North Am 1993; 20:217–246

7. Motzer RJ, Bander NH, Nanus DM. Renal-cell carcinoma. N Engl J Med 1996; 335(12): 865–874

8. Parkin DM, Whelan SL, Ferlay J, Raymond L, Young J (eds). Cancer incidence in five continents, Vol. VII. IARC Scientific Publications No. 143. Lyon: International Agency for Research on Cancer, 1997

9. Gould A, Muir CS, Sharp L. Prognosis and survival in prostate cancer. In: Epidemiology of prostate disease, Garraway M (ed.). Berlin: Springer-Verlag, 1995

10. Linehan WM, Lerman MI, Zbar B. Identification of the von Hippel–Lindau (VHL) gene, its role in renal cancer. JAMA 1995; 273:564–570

11. Brauch H, Weirich G, Hornauer M, Storkel S, Wohl T, Bruning T. Trichlorethylene exposure and specific somatic mutations in patients with renal cell carcinoma. JNCI 1999; 91(10):854–856

12. Yuan JM, Castelao J, Dominguez M, Ross R, Yu M. Hypertension, obesity and their medications in relation to renal cell carcinoma. Br J Cancer 1998; 77(9):1508–1513

13. Choyke PL, Glenn GM, Walther MM, Patronas NJ, Linehan WM, Zbar B. Von Hippel–Lindau disease: genetic, clinical and imaging features. Radiology 1995; 146:629–642

14. Bard RH, Lord B, Fromowitz F. Papillary adenocarcinoma of kidney. Urology 1982; 19:16–20

15. Akhtar M, Kardar H, Linjawi T, McClintock J, Ashraf M. Chromophobe cell carcinoma of the kidney. Am J Surg Pathol 1995; 19:1245–1256

16. Kennedy SM, Merino MJ, Linehan WM, Roberts JR, Robertson CN, Neumann RD. Collecting duct carcinoma of the kidney. Human Pathol 1990; 21:449–456

17. DeKernion JB, Mukamel E, Richie AW, Blyth B, Hannah J, Bohman R. Prognostic significance of

the DNA content of renal carcinoma. Cancer 1989; 64:1669–1673

18. Fuhrman SA, Lasky LC, Limas C. Prognostic significance of morphologic parameters in renal cell carcinoma. Am J Surg Pathol 1982; 6:655–663

19. Cherukuri S, Johenning P, Ram M. Systemic effects of hypernephroma. Urology 1977; 10(2): 93–97

20. Marshall F, Walsh P. Extra-renal manifestations of renal cell carcinoma. J Urol 1977; 117:439–440

21. Teigan EL, Newhouse JH. Imaging renal masses. Curr Opin Urol 2000; 10:421–427

22. Tsui K, Barbaric Z, Figlin R, deKernion J, Belldegrun A. Is adrenalectomy a necessary component of radical nephrectomy? UCLA experience with 511 radical nephrectomies. J Urol 2000; 163:437–441

23. Moll V, Becht, E, Zeigler M. Kidney preserving technique in renal cell tumors: indications, techniques and results in 152 patients. J Urol 1993; 150:319–323

24. Fergany AF, Hafez KS, Novick AC. Long term results of nephron sparing surgery for localized renal cell carcinoma: 10-year follow up. J Urol 2000; 163:442–445

25. Miller J, Fischer C, Freese R, Altmannsberger M, Weidner W. Nephron sparing surgery for renal cell carcinoma – is tumor size a suitable parameter or indication. Urology 1999; 54(6):988–992

26. Campbell SC, Krishnamurthi V, Chow G, Hale J, Myles J, Novick AC. Renal cryosurgery: experimental evaluation of treatment parameters. Urology 1998; 52:29–34

27. Khorsandi M, Foy RC, Chong W, et al. Preliminary experience with open renal cryoablation. J Urol 1999; 161(4):733A

28. Gill IS, Hobarg MG, Soble J, et al. Laparoscopic renal cryoablation in 32 patients. J Urol 1999; 161(4):729A

29. Nadasdy T, Bane BL, Silva FG. Adult renal disease. In: Diagnostic surgical pathology, 2nd edn, Sternberg C (ed.). New York; Raven Press, 1994

30. Yagoda A, Abi-rached B, Petrylak D. Chemotherapy for advanced renal-cell carcinoma. Semin Oncol 1995; 22:42–60

31. Harris DT. Hormonal therapy and chemotherapy of renal-cell carcinoma. Semin Oncol 1983; 10:422–430

32. Medical Research Council Renal Cancer Collaborators. Interferon-alpha and survival in metastatic renal carcinoma: early results of a randomised controlled trial. Lancet 1999; 353:14–17

33. Gleave ME, Elhilali M, Fradet Y, et al. Interferon gamma-1b compared with placebo in metastatic renal-cell carcinoma. N Engl J Med 1998; 338:1265–1271

34. Rosenberg SA, Yang JC, Topalian SL, et al. Treatment of 283 consecutive patients with metastatic melanoma or renal cell cancer using high-dose bolus interleukin-2. JAMA 1994; 271:907–913

35. Atzpodien J, Kirchner H, Hanninen EL. Interleukin-2 in combination with interferon-alpha and 5-fluorouracil for metastatic renal cell cancer. Eur J Cancer 1993; 29A:S6–8

36. Maher ER, Yates JR, Harries R, et al. Clinical features and natural history of von Hippel–Lindau disease. Q J Med 1990; 77:1151–1163

FURTHER READING

Cassileth BR, Zupkis RV, Sutton-Smith K, March V. Information and participation preferences among cancer patients. Ann Intern Med 1980; 92:1832–1836

Figlin R. Renal cell carcinoma: management of advanced disease. J Urol 1999; 161:381–387

Fuji A, Yui-en K, Ono H, Yamamoto K, Gohji K, Takenaka A. Preliminary results of the alternating administration of natural interferon-alpha and recombinant interferon-gamma for metastatic renal cell carcinoma. Br J Urol Int 1999; 84:399–404

Mickisch G, Carballido J, Hellsten S, Schulze H, Mensink H. Guidelines on renal cell cancer. Arnhem: EAU, 2001

7

Testis cancer

The stones are called in Latin testes, that is wit-
ness because they witness one to be a man, ask the
Pope else.... I need not tell you where they are
placed, for Every Boy that knows his right hand
from his left, knows that.... The use of the stones
is 1. To convert blood spirit into seed for the pro-
creation of man.... 2. They add heat, strength
and courage to the Body

Nicholas Culpeper[1]

GENERAL COMMENTARY

Testis cancer is generally a disease of younger males, and is the most common cancer between 20 and 40 years.[2] The overwhelming majority are germ cell tumours[3].

Testis cancer represents 5% of all urological tumours. In 1–2% of patients, the disease is bilateral.[3]

The treatment of testicular cancer has been a major success story in solid tumour oncology, and in the vast majority of patients, particularly where the disease has been arrested at an early stage, one can talk in terms of a probable cure to the patient, and cure rates of >95% are possible.[2]

INCIDENCE

The incidence of the disease is increasing, with an approximate increase of 15% between 1981 and 1990 (Table 7.1).[4]

International comparison of survival rates from testicular cancer (ICD-9 186) are shown in Table 7.2 and comparisons in Figure 7.1.

AETIOLOGICAL FACTORS

Cryptorchidism

Cryptorchidism is one of the most common disorders of childhood, with an incidence of 3.4% in full-term births. Defects of gonadotrophin production, androgen synthesis or action are associated with cryptorchidism. The longer a testis remains cryptorchid, the more likely it is to be histologically abnormal. Approximately 10% of testicular tumours arise in an undescended testis, and the undescended testis is between 35 and 48 times more likely to become malignant. The overall prevalence of carcinoma in situ is 1.7% in patients with cryptorchidism. The reason for an increase in cryptorchidism is imperfectly understood, but is thought to be due to maternal exposure to oestrogens. It is well recognised that an undescended testicle (UDT) has an increased risk of malignancy. For this reason, most urological surgeons recommend that orchidopexy is carried out before the age of 1. It is known that these testicles are often poorly developed, but what is not known is whether this procedure reduces the risk of subsequent development of cancer. Certainly, the testicle can be palpated more readily and an early cancer could be more readily detected. However, it is difficult to be sure that the risk of malignancy is reduced by this procedure, and the other testis remains at risk.[6]

Table 7.1 Age-standardised incidence rates and standard errors (SE) per 100,000 for cancer of testis (ICD-9: 186)[4]		
Country	**Incidence**	**SE**
Denmark	9.2	0.26
Germany: Eastern States	7.9	0.21
Austria, Tyrol	6.3	0.60
Germany: Saarland	6.1	0.46
US, Hawaii: White	5.9	0.77
UK, Scotland	5.8	0.21
US, SEER:[a] White	5.4	0.10
Czech Republic	5.2	0.14
Uruguay, Montevideo	4.8	0.50
Sweden	4.8	0.15
UK, England and Wales	4.6	0.08
Italy, Genoa	4.3	0.52
Poland, Warsaw City	4.1	0.37
The Netherlands	4.0	0.11
South Australia	4.0	0.32
Canada	3.8	0.07
Ecuador, Quito	3.5	0.35
France, Calvados	3.5	0.46
Ireland, Southern	3.4	0.52
US, Hawaii: Hawaiian	3.4	0.77
US, Hawaii: Japanese	3.0	0.73
Israel: all Jews	3.0	0.18
Argentina, Concordia	2.9	0.96
Peru, Lima	2.9	0.22
US, Hawaii: Filipino	2.7	1.21
US, Hawaii: Chinese	2.7	1.21
Yugoslavia, Vojvodina	2.6	0.23
Finland	2.5	0.13
Japan, Hiroshima	1.7	0.26
Spain, Zaragoza	1.5	0.27
Kuwait: non-Kuwaitis	1.5	0.51
Brazil, Goiania	1.3	0.33
Hong Kong	1.3	0.09
US, Puerto Rico	1.3	0.14
Singapore: Chinese	0.9	0.14
India, Bombay	0.9	0.07
Israel: non-Jews	0.8	0.22
Kuwait: Kuwaitis	0.8	0.29
Vietnam: Hanoi	0.7	0.16
Philippines, Manila	0.7	0.10
China, Shanghai	0.7	0.06
US, SEER: Black	0.7	0.11
Zimbabwe, Harare: African	0.6	0.38
Korea, Kangwa	0.3	0.31
Zimbabwe, Harare: European	–	–

[a]SEER = Surveillance, Epidemiology and End Results programme.

Table 7.2 Relative survival (%) at 5 years, all ages, patients diagnosed 1985–89[5]	
Country	**Relative survival (%)**
USA	95.7
Denmark	92.0
Finland	90.0
France	86.0
Germany	93.0
Italy	91.0
Netherlands	96.0
Spain	92.0
Sweden	92.0
England and Wales	90.0
Scotland	92.3

Declining sperm densities

It is believed that sperm densities have been declining in various countries, including the UK; the reasons are obscure. Paternal exposure to dioxins has been postulated.[7–9]

Timing of orchidopexy

Historically, surgery (orchidopexy) has varied in timing; some surgeons once preferred a conservative approach and delayed orchidopexy until after age 9. Currently, surgery is undertaken at the earliest opportunity, as histological changes in the undescended testis are detectable from the second year of life. Relationships are uncertain between the precise age at orchidopexy and the risk of subsequent cancer, as they also are with the nature of undescended testes (unilateral or bilateral) and associations with other congenital abnormalities. The same is true of possible psychological benefits of early as opposed to later intervention. Testicular cancer is not the only adverse outcome associated with testicular maldescent. Recent studies have revealed abnormal psycho-

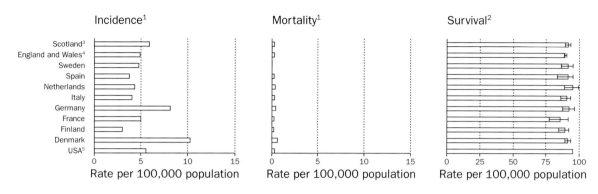

Incidence[1] Mortality[1] Survival[2]

Rate per 100,000 population / Rate per 100,000 population / Rate per 100,000 population

1 Age-standardised rates per 100,000 person-years at risk (World standard population) 1995.
2 Relative survival at 5 years, patients diagnosed 1985–89.

3 Scotland: survival, ages 15–99.
4 England and Wales: incidence 1993; mortality 1995; survival 1986–90 (ages 15–99).
5 USA (SEER, whites): incidence and mortality 1992–96; survival 1989–95.

Figure 7.1 International comparison of incidence, mortality and survival (with 95% CI) all ages.

sexual development and neurobehavioural abnormalities in older children with a history of cryptorchidism despite orchidopexy.[10,11]

Infertile males

The prevalence of testicular tumours in infertile men is 0.5%.[9]

Body size and testicular cancer

Patients who have a high body mass have a lower risk of testicular cancer, but taller patients have a positively associated risk.[12]

Genetic factors

Both polythelia and X-linked ichthyosis are documented as having an increased risk.

Recently, a gene on the X chromosome has been localised. This gene was localised to Xq27. Brothers of men with such tumours have an 8–10-fold risk of suffering similarly themselves. The proportion of families with undescended testicles linked to this locus was 73% compared with 26% of families without UDT.

These results provide evidence for a gene on chromosome Xq27 that may also predispose to UDT.[13]

PATHOLOGY

The cells of the testes may be divided into two groups. First, those of the germ cell elements,

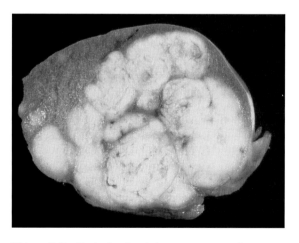

Figure 7.2 Typical cut potato appearance of seminoma specimen.

which produce the sperm and, secondly, the supporting elements in the seminiferous tubules, which are of two main types:

- Sertoli's cells
- Testosterone-producing Leydig's cells (interstitial cells).

Germ cell elements are far in excess of those other cells. Tumours of germ cell origin therefore account for a vast majority of testicular tumours.[14]

WORLD HEALTH ORGANIZATION CLASSIFICATION OF GERM CELL TUMOURS

The WHO classification of germ cell tumours is given in Box 7.1.

Box 7.1   WHO classification of germ cell tumours

Tumours of one histological type

Classical seminoma

Spermatocytic seminoma

Embryonal carcinoma

Yolk sac tumour (endodermal sinus tumour)

Polyembryoma

Choriocarcinoma

Pure teratoma

   Mature

   Immature

   With malignant transformation

Tumours of more than one histological type

Embryonal carcinoma and teratoma (teratocarcinoma)

Choriocarcinoma and any other type (specify type)

Other combinations (specify)

Adapted from Mostofi FK & Sobin LH.[14]

Teratomas

Teratoma is a germ cell neoplasm which shows de-differentiation from all three germ cell layers – namely, ectoderm, endoderm and mesoderm – and may therefore contain various cellular elements. Lymphomas may present as testicular swellings, especially in the elderly.

CLINICAL PRESENTATION

Early

Testes tumours usually present as a painless swelling within the scrotum, either as enlargement of the testicle as a whole or as a discrete lump within the testicle. Occasionally, the testis has been noted to have become smaller. Diagnostic confusion arises with inflammatory processes in the scrotum, and it is wise to remember that 31% present with pain and 15% present with inflammation.

Patients may occasionally complain of a dull ache, a dragging sensation felt in 29% of cases, or heaviness in the lower abdomen, but this is generally not the case. Patients can in rare circumstances present with a hydrocele.

Gynaecomastia can occasionally be the first manifestation of a teratoma, since they can elaborate many hormones and oestrogenic hormones cause the breast enlargement.

On examination, the swelling is generally hard and is part of the testis itself and not of the epididymis: 97% have a lump on examination at presentation.

An ultrasound of the scrotum shows a fairly typical solid appearance.

Late

Very occasionally, patients may present with symptoms due to metastases. These symptoms may be due to retroperitoneal lymph nodes causing back pain, obstruction of a ureter, occasionally renal failure and symptoms due to intrathoracic spread, such as cough or stridor. Occasionally, the patient may be noted to have lymph nodes in the neck.

CLASSIFICATION

The TNM (tumour, node, metastasis) staging system for testes cancer is shown in Table 7.3.

TUMOUR MARKERS

The three markers which are used routinely are β human chorionic gonadotrophin (β-HCG), alpha fetoprotein (AFP) and lactic acid dehydrogenase (LDH). Table 7.4 shows classification by the International Germ Cell Cancer Group and Table 7.5 shows staging based on serum tumour markers. A rise in AFP is associated with yolk sac or embryonal elements. Pure seminomas do not increase these markers. It is imperative that these blood tests are taken prior to any surgery.

SCREENING

It would be impracticable to screen for this relatively rare tumour. The optimal approach is to carry out public awareness programmes and encourage all males to report any new lumps or changes over time. Testicular self-examination should be encouraged on a monthly basis. It is wise to emphasise the curability of the disease at an early stage. This information is also given with benefit to women who may encourage their partners to seek help.[15,16]

DIAGNOSIS

The diagnosis is first made clinically. The presence of a hard area within the substance of the

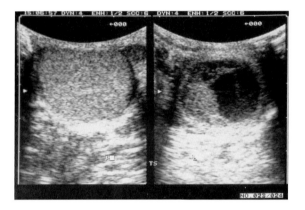

Figure 7.3 Ultrasound of both testes. The left-hand image of the right testis is homogeneous and normal. The image of the left testis demonstrates necrotic testicular teratoma.

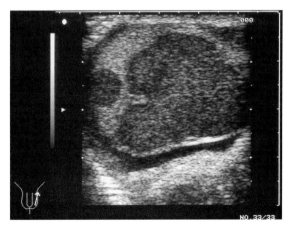

Figure 7.4 Left testicular ultrasound demonstrating multinodular seminoma.

Table 7.3	TNM classification of testes cancer
Stage	**Finding**
PTis	Intratubular
pT1	Testis and epididymis, no vascular/lymphatic invasion
pT2	Testis and epididymis with vascular/lymphatic invasion or tunica vaginalis
pT3	Spermatic cord
pT4	Scrotum
N1	<2 cm
N2	>2–5 cm
N3	>5 cm
M1a	Non-regional lymph node or pulmonary metastasis
M1b	Non-pulmonary visceral metastasis

Table 7.4   IGCCC prognostic grouping

Teratoma (NSGCT)	Seminoma
Good prognosis with all of:	
Testis/retroperitoneal primary	Any primary site
No non-pulmonary visceral metastases	No non-pulmonary visceral metastases
AFP < 1000 ng/ml	Normal AFP
HCG > 5000 iu/L	Any HCG
LDH < 1.5 upper limit of normal	Any LDH
56% of teratomas 5-year survival 92%	90% of seminomas 5-year survival 86%
Intermediate prognosis:	
Testis/retroperitoneal primary	Any primary site
No non-pulmonary visceral metastases	Non-pulmonary visceral metastases[a]
and any of:	
AFP > 1000 and <10,000 ng/ml and/or	Normal AFP
HCG > 5000 and <50,000 iu/L and/or	Any HCG
LDH > 1.5 normal < 10 normal	Any LDH
28% of teratomas 5-year survival 80%	10% of seminomas 5-year survival 73%
Poor prognosis with any of:	
Mediastinal primary or non-pulmonary visceral metastases	*No patients in this group*
AFP > 10,000 ng/L and/or	
HCG > 50,000 iu/L and/or	
LDH > 10 normal	
16% of teratomas 5-year survival 48%	

[a] Non-pulmonary visceral metastases refers to liver, bone, brain and skin.[13]
AFP = alpha fetoprotein; LDH = lactic acid dehydrogenase; HCG = human chorionic gonadotrophin.

Table 7.5   American Joint Committee on Cancer-serum Tumour Markers (S stage)

Stage	Serum marker		
SX	Serum markers not available		
S0	Serum marker study levels within normal limits		
	LDH	HCG (ml/U/ml)	AFP (ng/ml)
S1	<1.5 × N	and <5000	and <1000
S2	1.5–10 × N	or 5000–50,000	or 1000–10,000
S3	>10 × N	or >50,000	or >10,000

N indicates the upper limit or normal for the LDH assay. AFP = alpha fetoprotein; LDH = lactic acid dehydrogenase; HCG = human chorionic gonadotrophin.

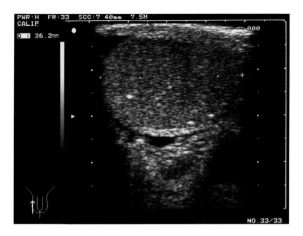

Figure 7.5 Right testicular ultrasound demonstrating microlithiasis in contralateral testis (same patient).

testicle is usually made by the clinician. The patient may have noticed it, although this is by no means always the case.

Ultrasonography has a near 100% sensitivity for detecting testicular tumours,[16] which are visualised mainly as hypoechoic areas.

Testicular microlithiasis can be seen in 45% of cases of testicular cancer[17] and its significance is uncertain. As an isolated finding, it is probably advisable to repeat ultrasound scans although the information is less than clear.[18]

Biopsy of the testis through the scrotum is not recommended.

SURGICAL MANAGEMENT OF TESTICULAR CANCER

Primary treatment – orchiectomy (OPCS code N0680)

The initial surgical management involves obtaining informed consent, to explore the testicle and remove it.

Staging
The patient may have a preoperative chest X-ray and, occasionally, an ultrasound of the abdomen or a computed tomography (CT)

scan. However, the patient is normally given a place on the next available surgical list.

Cross-matching
Cross-matching is not usually necessary.

Heparin
Heparin, 5000 units given subcutaneously pre-operatively, until the patient is ambulant.

Surgical anatomy of the inguinal canal and scrotum

It continues to be traditional to operate on tumours through the inguinal canal. The canal is an oblique slit, starting at the deep inguinal ring and contains the spermatic cord. Its anterior wall is the external oblique aponeurosis, but its floor is that of the lower edge of the inguinal ligament. The roof of the canal is formed by the internal oblique and transversus abdominis muscles and posteriorly, the wall of the canal is formed by the conjoint tendon medially and the transversalis fascia laterally.

The spermatic cord is exposed by incising the external oblique muscle laterally from the superficial inguinal ring. The cord is gently mobilised by sharp and blunt dissection and can be clamped at an early stage in the procedure. Some surgeons put double clamps on. It is important to divide the spermatic cord as high as possible, ensuring that the proximal end does not retract into the abdomen. Once the cord is divided, the residual cord is transfixually ligated with an absorbable suture, and if there is any doubt as to the effectiveness of this suture, a second suture should be applied.

The testicle is carefully delivered up through the canal, remembering that it may have developed blood supply from the scrotum. It is important to ensure that the scrotum is not 'buttonholed' and thus opened inadvertently.

The cord and testicle are explored through the groin. It is recommended that a soft clamp be placed round the cord, prior to mobilisation of the testicle, to minimise potential blood spread of the tumour during mobilisation.

Where there is reasonable doubt, a frozen-section diagnosis of tumour may be made but, in general, the testis is removed along with the cord, transfixing the cord at the highest level practicable at the deep ring, taking care not to let the vessels retract through the deep ring before being suitably ligated, generally with a transfixion suture.

Sometimes, the testicle has to be opened to locate a tumour. Excision biopsy of an intratesticular lesion can damage the blood supply of the testis if it is not removed, and this risk needs to be explained to the patient where relevant.

Occasionally, the patient may wish for the prosthesis to be inserted and this can be done at the time of operation, although generally the patients are too scared to think about this. Nonetheless, this should be offered.

Specimens are sent to the Pathology Department. In the recovery period, it is usually a convenient time for CT scans to be undertaken.

FERTILITY

The patient may be aware of difficulties with fertility and should be offered sperm storage procedures prior to any chemotherapy or radiotherapy. It should be realised, however, that many of these patients are either unable to produce a specimen or the sperm sample at the time of surgery is of poor quality. At the time of orchidectomy for testicular cancer, about half the patients have abnormal sperm concentrations.[19,20]

THE CONTRALATERAL TESTIS

Biopsy of the 'uninvolved opposite testis' should be considered (OPCS code N1340, N134). This may be deferred until after sperm storage. Approximately 5% of men with testis cancer have carcinoma in situ (CIS) on the contralateral side. Progression to carcinoma occurs in 50–100% of patients with CIS.

An identifiable high-risk group exists:

- the remaining testis of small volume (<16 ml)
- low sperm count
- ultrasound abnormality of remaining testis
- patients <30 years
- history of maldescent

Biopsy procedure

After informed consent, and under general anaesthetic, an open large needle biopsy is taken without crushing the specimen. It is recommended that 0.3–1.0 cm be sent for histology.

Ideally, two specimens should be sent: one in Bouin's fluid, and the other in formal saline.

The pathologist will determine the presence of CIS, the degree of spermatogenesis and whether there is atrophy of the seminiferous tubules.

Management of CIS in the contralateral testis

If CIS is demonstrated in the contralateral testis, radiotherapy to the testis should be discussed. This prevents CIS progressing (typically, 20 Gy is given in 10 fractions over 2 weeks). Fertility is lost, but potency remains.

CLASSIFICATION OF RISK FACTORS FOR TESTICULAR CANCER

Epidemiological

- Cryptorchidism
- Klinefelter's syndrome
- Familial history
- Contralateral tumour
- Tin
- Infertility.

Pathological (for stage 1)

- Histopathological type
- Tumour size
- Vascular/lymphatic peritumoral invasion.

Clinical (for metastatic disease)

- Primary location
- Elevation of tumour marker levels
- Presence of non-pulmonary visceral metastasis (only clinical predictive factor for metastatic disease in seminoma).

EUROPEAN ASSOCIATION OF UROLOGY (EAU) GUIDELINES

EAU guidelines are given in Box 7.2.

Box 7.2   EAU guidelines on diagnosis and staging of testicular cancer

1. Physical examination may be sufficient for the diagnosis of testicular cancer.
2. Testicular ultrasound is mandatory when a tumour is clinically suspected but the examination of the scrotum is normal or if there is any doubt about the clinical findings in the scrotum.
3. Pathological examination of the testis is necessary to confirm the diagnosis and define the local extension (pT category).
4. Serum determination of tumour markers (AFP, β-HCG, LDH) must be performed before and after orchidectomy for staging and prognostic reasons.
5. Retroperitoneal, mediastinal and supraclavicular nodes and visceral state have to be assessed in testicular cancer. In seminoma, a chest CT scan is not necessary if abdominal nodes are negative.

CHEMOTHERAPY FOR TESTICULAR CANCER

Tumour markers should be repeated after orchidectomy. Where the markers remain high, there is unequivocal evidence of persistent disease. It is essential at this stage that consultation with an experienced oncologist take place.

MANAGEMENT OF EARLY (STAGE 1) DISEASE

This is defined as no residual disease following orchidectomy. There is no evidence of metastatic disease on clinical examination, and a normal CT scan of the chest, abdomen and pelvis and normal postoperative tumour markers.

Management of stage 1 seminoma

At present there is no reliable marker for seminoma, and there is a 15% probability of returns within 3 years. This compares with a 3% risk of relapse after adjuvant retroperitoneal radiation. Surveillance should not therefore be considered acceptable in patients where fertility is of a particular issue.

Radiotherapy is carried out to the para-aortic nodes and to any pelvic lymph nodes which are involved, as determined radiologically or surgically. Normally, unless there are risk factors for pelvic node disease, the para-aortic nodes are radiated using parallel opposed fields from T10–LV5 and a dose of 30 Gy in 15 fractions is a typical dose.

Stage 1 seminoma with the risk of pelvic node disease

Where there has been previous inguinal scrotal surgery, the radiation fields are widened to include the ipsilateral pelvic nodes. The failure rate following this is 6%.

Where risk factors of pelvic nodal disease exist, prophylactic para-aortic irradiation is carried out; once again, a dose of 30 Gy in 15 fractions over 3 weeks would be a typical dosage.

If inadvertently a scrotal incision has been used, the advice at present is that the scrotum should only be included in the radiotherapy field if it was felt that there was a high risk of tumour contamination.

Management of stage 1 teratoma and mixed seminoma/teratoma

There is a relapse rate of 30% in patients treated by surveillance. The most important histological predictors of relapse are invasion of the blood vessels or lymphatic invasion, increasing the risk of relapse to 40%.

Because these tumours are curable, the patients with stage 1 teratomas or mixed seminoma teratomas can be managed initially by surveillance following removal of the primary testicular tumour.

Common sense must be used in following up patients and advocating surveillance. Where there is a risk of patients defaulting, there is a much stronger argument for initial treatment. Patients are seen monthly, and clinical examination and markers carried out. A chest X-ray is performed monthly. A CT of the chest and abdomen is performed at 3, 6, 9 and 12 months.

After 1 year of disease-free surveillance, CT scans are carried out at 18 and 24 months, but the patient is seen every 2 months.

The SIGN guidelines recommend, subsequently, that the patient should be seen 3-monthly for the 3rd year, 6-monthly until the 5th year and annually thereafter for 10 years. At each visit, serum markers and chest X-ray are performed.

Pelvic nodal disease is associated with risk factors such as previous scrotal or inguinal surgery, previous retroperitoneal surgery/irradiation, invasive tumour through the tunica albuginea and bulky abdominal nodes.

Adjuvant chemotherapy

Patients should be entered into studies. Standard chemotherapy would involve platinum-based chemotherapy, i.e. bleomycin, etoposide and cisplatin (BEP). Adjuvant chemotherapy can also be used in patients who do not wish surveillance and in whom it is felt that surveillance is inappropriate. It is also recommended that the chemotherapy be offered to patients with evidence of blood

Table 7.6	Metastatic seminoma
Stage	**Treatment**
IIa	Radiation therapy to para-aortic and ipsilateral lymph nodes
IIb	Chemotherapy or radiotherapy as initial treatment
IIc	Cisplatin-based chemotherapy initially
IId	Cisplatin-based chemotherapy initially
III	Cisplatin-based chemotherapy
IV	Cisplatin-based chemotherapy

vessel or lymphatic invasion. Normally, two courses of BEP chemotherapy are given.

MANAGEMENT OF METASTATIC DISEASE

Metastatic seminoma is divided into groups A, B, C and D. These are divided on the basis of the bulk of retroperitoneal disease. The stages and treatment of metastatic seminoma are shown in Table 7.6.

Management of metastatic teratoma

Standard therapy for patients with metastatic teratoma would typically be four cycles of chemotherapy, based on bleomycin, etoposide and cisplatin (BEP). There is debate as to whether a full four courses are required, and it is essential that all decisions are made by experienced oncologists, in a centre experienced in management of germ cell tumours.

Normally, cisplatin should be used and carboplatin should only be used where cisplatin is contraindicated. BEP is also used for patients with intermediate and poor-risk germ cell tumours as initial treatment.

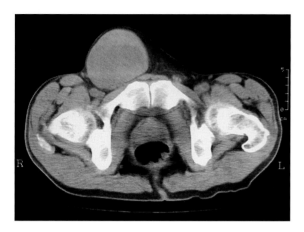

Figure 7.6 CT image of pelvis demonstrating right testicular teratoma in an undescended inguinal testis.

Treatment of residual masses after chemotherapy

Seminoma

It would be unusual to recommend resection of residual seminoma because of the difficulty in removing the tumour, due to problems in finding clear tissue planes and tissue infiltration beyond resection margins.

Teratoma

Remaining masses may contain viable tumour after chemotherapy, despite markers becoming normal. It is important to be able to differentiate between residual tumour and fibrosis or tumour necrosis. This differentiation is carried out by surgical removal. The surgery aims to clear all the residual mass and associated abnormal tissue.

Retroperitoneal lymph node dissection (RPLND) OPCS code T8540, T854)

This surgery is highly specialised and is increasingly the province of the specialised uro-oncologist, with a particular interest in this technique. Incisions used may be either thoracoabdominal incisions or midline incisions from the sternum to pubis. The advantage of the thoracoabdominal incision is that there is said to be a lower instance of postoperative obstruction.

All lymph node tissue between the ureters from the renal vessels to the bifurcation of the common iliac vessels is removed. Nephrectomy is occasionally necessary.

RPLND is associated with significant morbidity.

Standard dissection leads almost inevitably to loss of ejaculation. This is due to damage to the sympathetic nerve fibres. In view of this, a modification of this technique has been introduced to remove only the lymph nodes on the same side as the tumour and below the inferior mesenteric artery. This generally leaves the patient with ejaculatory ability, which is important, since most of the patients are young.

Where the resected specimen shows residual tumour, further chemotherapy should be considered.

Patients with seminoma, who have residual masses following chemotherapy may be managed by a policy of observation rather than radiotherapy.

Relapsed disease

A combined approach is required, but surgery is the main treatment for relapsed teratoma.

Where central nervous system (CNS) involvement is found, surgical resection of accessible CNS lesions should be considered and radiotherapy may be given as part of the treatment option or on a curative or palliative basis. The patient will then be offered chemotherapy, usually based round cisplatin. At follow-up, CT scans may show the patient to have residual disease. After a varying number of cycles of chemotherapy, usually after three, re-staging occurs. If residual lymph nodes occur, then the patient should be referred to a surgeon experienced in RPLND.

PROGNOSTIC FACTORS

Prognostic factors in testicular cancer:

- histological prognostic factors – percentage of embryonal carcinoma within the primary tumour

- vascular invasion of testicular veins
- serum tumour markers – AFP
- β-HCG
- LDH.

TESTICULAR CANCER – CASE HISTORY 1
(patient permission obtained)

A 30-year-old male developed a painful swelling of his left groin, which was noted on examination. An ultrasound suggested a testicular tumour in an undescended testis.

At surgery, a left testicular tumour was noted in the inguinal canal. This was removed through a groin incision, ligating the cord at the internal ring. His AFP prior to surgery was 11,400 u/ml, but his β-HCG was less than 1. A CT scan was carried out to stage the tumour. The AFP dropped 2 days postoperatively to 11,300 u/ml and then 3 weeks later had dropped to 5200 u/ml. His CT scan showed no definite evidence of metastatic disease in the abdomen or chest.

At review, his wound was satisfactory and his markers continued to fall. Because his markers were so high, however, it was felt that he should be treated with cisplatin-based chemotherapy.

Sperm storage was arranged and a staging CT scan was carried out. He was entered into the Medical Research Council – Treatment of Good Prognosis Germ Cell Cancer Trial. The CT scan showed that he had a 3 cm para-aortic lymph node mass. He was then treated with bleomycin, etoposide and cisplatin.

The patient was warned that the treatment was moderately myelosuppressive and that he was told to contact the ward if there were any problems.

He received four courses of treatment and tolerated his chemotherapy well. He finally developed some tiredness and feelings of being hot. He was found to be slightly neutropenic. No specific treatment was required. Specifically, he had no complaints of mucositis or indigestion.

A subsequent CT scan showed regression of the para-aortic lymphadenopathy, but he still had two nodes of 1.5 cm in diameter.

He was referred for excision of lymph nodes. Because of his size, he needed an extra-peritoneal thoracoabdominal approach to the tumour.

Histology confirmed no evidence of metastatic teramona, and the patient went back into surveillance. A chest X-ray showed continuing raised left hemi-diaphragm, but nothing else of note. His tumour markers remained low and his chest X-ray was normal. There is no evidence of recurrent disease and one would expect him to have an excellent prognosis.

TESTICULAR CANCER – CASE HISTORY 2
(patient permission obtained)

A 22-year-old man had a 3-week history of a left testicular lump. On examination, he was noted to have a 3 cm × 4 cm mass at the upper pole of the left testis. An ultrasound confirmed the appearance of a testicular carcinoma.

At operation there was a definite intratesticular mass in the upper pole, but no evidence of involvement of the cord structures. He had AFP and HCG taken prior to surgery and a staging CT scan of his abdomen and pelvis was obtained. His preoperative AFP was 135 u/ml and HCG was 10,000 u/ml and he was referred to the clinical oncologists. Sperm storage was arranged.

His CT scan showed metastatic disease in the para-aortic nodes, although it appeared to be of a small volume. He received a course of bleomycin, etoposide and cisplatin, which was uneventful. He was warned that the chemotherapy would cause alopecia, nausea, lethargy and moderately severe myelosuppression. He had been made aware of the risk of infection between courses of chemotherapy and given a contact number to ring. He was told at that stage that his prognosis was excellent and that he would have a greater than 90% chance of cure.

Since he was in full-time education, his studies had to be interrupted by this.

He completed four cycles of chemotherapy and a follow-up CT scan was arranged. This showed some residual lymphadenopathy in the abdomen, in the para-aortic lymph nodes, measuring 1 cm in diameter but extending over

5 cm in length in the craniocaudal direction. An RPLND was performed.

Subsequently, his AFP and HCG were well within normal limits. There remained one or two tiny nodes seen on repeat CT scan and his chest X-rays were normal. The tiny para-aortic lymph nodes remained static and he is being followed up expectantly.

TESTICULAR TUMOURS IN CHILDREN

General testicular tumours account for 2% of all paediatric solid tumours and paediatric testicu- lar tumours account for 2% of all testicular tumours.[21]

Incidence

Peak incidence is at 2 years. Children appear to have a higher incidence of benign tumours.

Presentation

Painless scrotal swelling.

Table 7.7 Classification of prepubertal testis tumours (from Kaplan[21])	
Stage	**Type**
I	Germ cell tumours:
	yolk-sac tumour
	teratoma
	teratocarcinoma
	seminoma
II	Gonadal stromal tumours:
	Leydig's cell
	Sertoli's cell
	intermediate forms
III	Gonadoblastoma
IV	Tumours of supporting tissues:
	fibroma
	leiomyoma
	haemangioma
V	Lymphomas and leukaemias
VI	Tumour-like lesions:
	epidermoid cyst
	hyperplastic nodule attributable to congenital adrenal hyperplasia
VII	Secondary tumours
VIII	Tumours of adnexa

Table 7.8 Intergroup staging system for testicular germ cell tumours	
Stage	**Extent of disease**
I	Limited to testis (testes), completely resected by high inguinal orchidectomy; no clinical, radiographic, or histologic evidence of disease beyond the testes; tumour markers normal after appropriate half-life decline (AFP, 5 days; β-HCG, 16 hours). Patients with normal or unknown tumour markers at diagnosis must have a negative ipsilateral retroperitoneal node sampling to confirm stage I disease
II	Transscrotal orchidectomy; microscopic disease in scrotum or high in spermatic cord (<5 cm from proximal end); retroperitoneal lymph node involvement (<2 cm) and/or persistently elevated or increased tumour markers
III	Retroperitoneal lymph node involvement (<2 cm), but no visceral or extra-abdominal involvement
IV	Distant metastases, including liver

AFP = alpha fetoprotein; β-HCG = β-human chorionic gonadotrophin.

Classification

There is no fully accepted classification of testicular tumours in children. A classification system for prepubertal testis tumours is given in Table 7.7.

Staging

An intergroup staging system for testicular germ cell tumours is shown in Table 7.8.

Metastases

Germ cell tumours metastasise to the lungs in 20% of patients and 5% have retroperitoneal lymph nodes. It should be noted that seminoma is extremely rare in children.[21]

REFERENCES

1. Culpeper N. A directory for midwives. London: Peter and Edward Cole, 1660
2. Dearnaley D, Huddart RA, Horwich A. Managing testicular cancer. Br Med J 2001; 322: 1583–1588
3. Laguna P, Pizzocaro G, Klepp O, Algaba F, Kisbenedek L, Leiva O. Guidelines on testicular cancer. Arnhem, the Netherlands: European Association of Urology, 2001
4. Parkin DM, Whelan SL, Ferlay J, Raymond L, Young J (eds). Cancer incidence in five continents, Vol. VII. IARC Publications No 143, Lyons: International Agency for Research on Cancer, 1997
5. Gould A, Muir CS, Sharp L. Prognosis and survival in prostate cancer. In: Epidemiology of prostate disease, Garraway M (ed.). Berlin: Springer-Verlag, 1995
6. Abratt RP, Reddi VB, Sarembock LA. Testicular cancer and cryptorchidism. Br J Urol 1992; 70:656
7. Martin DC, Menck HR. The undescended testis: management after puberty. J Urol 1975; 114:77–79
8. Irvine S, Cawood E, Richardson D, Macdonald E, Aitken J. Evidence of deteriorating semen quality in the UK: birth cohort study in 577 men in Scotland over 11 years. Br Med J 1996; 312: 467–471
9. Moccarelli P, Gerthoux PM, Ferrari E, et al. Paternal concentrations of dioxin and sex ratio of offspring. Lancet 2000; 355:1858–1863
10. Giwercman A, von der Maase H, Skakkebaek NE. Epidemiological and clinical aspects of carcinoma in-situ of the testis. Eur Urol 1993; 23:104–114
11. Pierik FH, Dohle GR, van Muiswinkel JM, Vreeburg JTM, Weber RFA. Is routine scrotal ultrasound in infertile men advantageous? J Urol 1999; 162:1618–1620
12. Acrae O, Ekbom A, Sparen P. Body size in testicular cancer. JNCI 2000; 92(13):1093–1096
13. Rapley EA, Crockford GP, Teare D, et al. Localization to Xq27 of a susceptibility gene for testicular germ-cell tumours. Nat Genet 2000; 24(2):197–200
14. Mostofi FK, Sobin LH. International histological classification of tumours of testes (No. 16). Geneva: World Health Organization, 1977
15. Royal College of Radiologists in partnership with Scottish Intercollegiate Guidelines Network. Guidelines for the management of adult testicular germ cell tumours. London: Royal College of Radiologists Clinical Oncology Network, 1999
16. Thornhill JA, Conroy RM, Kelly DG, Walsh A, Fennelly JJ, Fitzpatrick JM. Public awareness of testicular cancer and the value of self-examination. Br Med J 1986; 293:480–481
17. Dohle GR, Schroder FH. Ultrasonographic assessment of the scrotum. Lancet 2000; 356:1625–1626
18. Hobarth K, Susani M, Szabo N, Kratzik C. Incidence of testicular microlithiasis. Urology 1992; 40:464–467
19. Furness PD, Husmann DA, Brock JW, et al. Multi-institutional study of testicular microlithiasis in childhood: a benign or pre-malignant condition? J Urol 1998; 160:151–154
20. Kuczyk M, Machtens S, Bokemeyer C, Schultheiss D, Jonas U. Sexual function and fertility after treatment of testicular cancer. Curr Opin Urol 2000; 10:473–474
21. Kaplan GW. Testicular tumours in children. AUA Update Series, Lesson 12, Vol. 2, 1983

FURTHER READING

Bosl GJ, Motzer RJ. Medical progress: testicular germ cell cancer (a review article). N Engl J Med 1997; 337:242–263
Chilvers C, Saunders M, Bliss J, Nicholls J, Horwich A. Influence of delay in diagnosis on prognosis in

testicular teratoma. Br J Cancer 1989; 59:126–128.

Cooper ER. The histology of the retained testis in the human subject at different ages and its comparison with the testis. J Anat 1929; 64:5

Cullen MH, Billingham LJ, Cook J, Woodroffe CM. Management preferences in stage I non seminomatous germ cell tumors of the testes: an investigation among patients, controls and oncologists. Br J Cancer 1996; 74:1487–1491.

De Wit R. Treatment of disseminated non-seminomatous testicular cancer: the European experience. Sem Surg Oncol 1999; 17:250–256

Donohue JP, Einhorn L, Williams S. Cytoreductive surgery for metastatic testis cancer: considerations of timing and extent. J Urol 1980; 123: 876–880

Einhorn L, Donohue J. Cis-diamminedichloroplatinum, vinblastine, and bleomycin combination chemotherapy in disseminated testicular cancer. Ann Intern Med 1977; 87:293–298

Fordham MV, Mason MD, Blackmore C, Hendry WF, Horwich A. Management of the contralateral testis in patients with testicular germ cell cancer. Br J Urol 1990; 65:290–293.

Freedman LS, Jones WG, Peckham MJ, et al. Histopathology in the prediction of relapse of patients with stage I testicular teratoma treated by orchidectomy alone. Lancet 1987; ii:294–298

Gimmi C, Sonntag R, Brunner K. Adjuvant treatment of high risk clinical stage I testicular carcinoma with cisplatin, bleomycin and vinblastine or etoposide. Proc Am Soc Clin Oncol 1990; 9:140 (abstr)

Giwercman A, Maase H von der, Skakkebaek NE. Epidemiological and clinical aspects of carcinoma in situ of the testis. Eur Urol 1993; 23:104–114

Hendry WF, A'Hern RP, Hetherington JW, Peckham MJ, Dearnaley DP, Horwich A. Para-aortic lymphadenopathy after chemotherapy for metastatic non-seminomatous germ cell tumours: prognostic value and therapeutic benefit. Br J Urol 1993; 71:208–213

Higby DJ, Wallace HJ, Albert DJ, Wallace JF. Diamminedichloroplatinum: a phase I study showing responses in testicular and other tumours. Cancer 1974; 33:1219–1225

Lashley DB, Lowe BA. A rational approach to managing stage I non seminomatous germ cell cancer. Urol Clin N Am 1999; 25(3):405–423

Peckham MJ, Barrett A, Husband J, Hendry WF. Orchidectomy alone in testicular stage I non-seminomatous germ cell tumours. Lancet 1982; ii:678–680

Pont J, Holtl W, Kosak D. Risk adapted treatment choice in stage I non-seminomatous testicular germ cell cancer by regarding vascular invasion in the primary tumor. A prospective trial. J Clin Oncol 1990; 8:16–20.

Rajfer J. Congenital anomalies of the testis and scrotum. In: Campbell's urology, 7th edn, Walsh PC, Retik AB, Vaughan ED, Wein AJ (eds). Philadelphia: WB Saunders, 1997

Ray B, Hajdu SI, Whitmore WF Jr. Distribution of retroperitoneal lymph nodal metastases in testicular germ cell tumours. Cancer 1974; 33:340–348

Scorer CG, Farrington GH. Congenital deformities of the testis and epididymis. New York: Appleton-Century-Crofts, 1971

Skakkebaek NE. Possible carcinoma in situ of the testis. Lancet 1972; 1:516

Skakkebaek NE, Berthelsen JG, Visfeldt J. Clinical aspects of testicular carcinoma in situ. Int J Andrology 1981; (suppl 4):153–162

Snyder HM, D'Angio GJ, Evans AE, Raney RB. Paediatric oncology. In: Campbell's urology, 7th edn, Walsh PC, Retick AB, Vaughan ED, Wein AJ (eds). Philadelphia: WB Saunders, 1998

Steyerberg EW, Keizer HJ, Fossa SD, et al. Prediction of residual retroperitoneal mass histology after chemotherapy for metastatic nonseminomatous germ cell tumour: multivariate analysis of individual patient data from six study groups. J Clin Oncol 1995; 13:1177–1187

Studer UE, Fey MF, Calderoni A, et al. Adjuvant chemotherapy after orchiectomy in high risk patients with clinical stage. Eur Urol 1993; 23:444–449

Von der Maase H, Giwercman A, Skakkebaek NE. Radiation treatment of carcinoma-in-situ of testis. Lancet 1986; i:624–625.

Williams SD, Stablein DM, Einhorn LH, et al. Immediate adjuvant chemotherapy versus observation with treatment at relapse in pathologic stage II testicular cancer. N Engl J Med 1987; 317:1433–1438

8

Penile cancer

The functioning role of the penis is as well established as that of any other organ of the body. ... The organ has been venerated, reviled, and misrepresented with intent in art, literature, and legend through the centuries.

Masters & Johnson[1]

GENERAL COMMENTARY

Penile cancer is a rare cancer. The majority of penile cancers are squamous cell carcinomas. Melanomata and basal cell carcinomata are excessively rare due to lack of exposure to sunlight.

AETIOLOGY

The disease is said to be related to poor hygiene. It is extremely rare in men who are circumcised at an early age, but circumcision at a later age does not alter the risk. Poor genital hygiene leads to a build up of smegma – debris from sebaceous glands. Smegma is composed of 26% fat, 13% protein, hydrocarbons and steroids.[2]

There is believed to be an association with human papillomavirus (HPV) infection. There are around 80 types of HPV, and two-thirds cause genital infection. Up to 30% of male partners of women with severe cervical dysplasia or CIS of the female genital tract have dysplasia or CIS of the penis, but the rates seem lower in circumcised US males.[2,3]

SCREENING

Screening is not practicable.

INCIDENCE

Exclusively male. Incidence rates, by country, are compared in Table 8.1.

International comparison of survival rates from penile and other male genital organs cancer (ICD-9 187) are shown in Table 8.2.

PROGNOSTIC FACTORS

- Lymph node status
- T stage
- Tumour grade (Broders')
- Vascularity
- Microvascular invasion.

PRESENTATION

The disease presents almost always as a localised lesion: about 50% present on the glans, 20% present on the prepuce, 10% on the glans and prepuce, 5% on the coronal sulcus and less than 2% on the shaft. The tumour may present as:

- a red area on the penis
- a hardened area on the penis
- an exophytic growth on the glans penis
- priapism (where there is metastatic involvement).

Table 8.1 Age-standardised incidence rates and standard errors (SE) per 100,000 for cancer of penis (ICD-9 187)[4]

Country	Incidence	SE
Zimbabwe, Harare: African	2.8	0.91
US, Puerto Rico	2.5	0.18
Vietnam, Hanoi	2.3	0.32
Brazil, Goiania	2.1	0.48
India, Bombay	1.6	0.12
US, Hawaii: Filipino	1.5	0.59
UK, Scotland	1.2	0.08
France, Calvados	1.0	0.23
Germany, Eastern States	1.0	0.07
Germany, Saarland	1.0	0.16
Singapore: Chinese	1.0	0.15
Poland, Warsaw City	1.0	0.16
Zimbabwe, Harare: European	0.9	0.90
Uruguay, Montevideo	0.9	0.20
US, SEER:[a] Black	0.9	0.13
Czech Republic	0.9	0.05
Denmark	0.9	0.07
Ireland, Southern	0.8	0.23
Italy, Genoa	0.9	0.17
The Netherlands	0.8	0.05
Spain, Zaragoza	0.8	0.16
Sweden	0.9	0.05
UK, England and Wales	0.9	0.03
Peru, Lima	0.8	0.14
Canada	0.8	0.03
Philippines, Manila	0.7	0.12
US, SEER: White	0.7	0.03
Yugoslavia, Vojvodina	0.7	0.11
Argentina, Concordia	0.6	0.40
Hong Kong	0.6	0.06
Korea, Kangwa	0.6	0.42
Austria, Tyrol	0.6	0.18
Ecuador, Quito	0.6	0.19
China, Shanghai	0.5	0.05
US, Hawaii: Japanese	0.3	0.14
US, Hawaii: Hawaiian	0.3	0.28
Finland	0.5	0.05
South Australia	0.5	0.11
Israel: all Jews	0.2	0.05
Israel: non-Jews	0.2	0.08
Kuwait: non-Kuwaitis	0.2	0.11
US, Hawaii: White	0.2	0.14
Japan, Hiroshima	0.06	0.14
Kuwait: Kuwaitis	–	–
US, Hawaii: Chinese	–	–

[a]SEER = Surveillance, Epidemiology and End Results programme.

Table 8.2 Relative survival (%) at 5 years, all ages, patients diagnosed 1985–89

Country	Relative survival (%)
England and Wales	83.0
France	80.0
Spain	77.0
Italy	75.0
Sweden	74.0
Denmark	71.0
Netherlands	70.0
Finland	69.0
Scotland	66.0
USA	n/a
Germany	n/a

Erythroplasia of Queyrat appears as a red discrete lesion on the glans penis and is carcinoma in situ (CIS).

Bowen's disease is a form of CIS occurring on follicle-bearing skin and thus is the equivalent of the shaft of the penis.

Lymph nodes may be present in the groin and, occasionally, this is due to coexistent infection. Where there is doubt about the diagnosis, an excision biopsy should be carried out. The

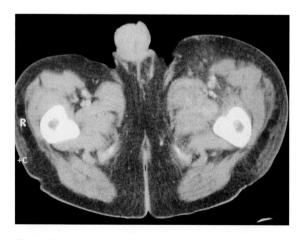

Figure 8.1 CT image of primary penile cancer.

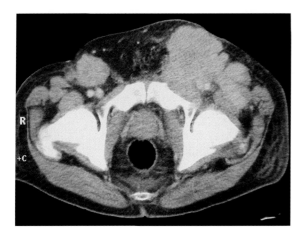

Figure 8.2 CT image of bilateral inguinal lymph node metastases from primary penile cancer (in same patient as Figure 8.1).

Table 8.3	TNM classification of penile cancer
Stage	**Finding**
Tis	In situ
Ta	Non-invasive verrucous carcinoma
T1	Subepithelial connective tissue
T2	Corpus spongiosum, cavernosum
T3	Urethra, prostate
T4	Other adjacent structures
N1	One superficial inguinal
N2	Multiple or bilateral superficial inguinal
N3	Deep inguinal or pelvic

presence of involved lymph nodes is the strongest prognostic feature.

About 20% of patients have hypercalcaemia, which is unrelated to metastases. The primary tumour or the involved lymph node may produce parathormone-like substances.

CLASSIFICATION

The TNM (tumour, node, metastasis) staging system for penile cancer is shown in Table 8.3.

TREATMENT

Treatment of primary lesion – biopsy

The primary lesion requires to be removed along with a 0.5 cm area of clearance.

It is usually appropriate to carry out circumcision.

The best forms of cure are carried out when a partial penectomy with a 2 cm margin is also undertaken. Ideally, a penile stump should allow voiding standing up.

Because of the destruction of tissue and disability produced, other forms of local treatment have been employed.

Mohs' microsurgery (MMS)[5]

First described by Mohs, this technique is used on small distal lesions on the glans penis. It can be carried out under local anaesthesia. Zinc chloride paste is applied to the area, which has been pretreated with dichloroacetic acid. Each layer is colour coded to allow subsequent identification.

Each layer can be removed in turn. Microscopy reveals layers of chemically fixed tissue; each layer can be examined in turn, and removal stopped when planes are obtained which are free from tumour.

Healing occurs by second intention, after sloughing of the deeper layers.

Laser surgery

Laser surgery using Nd:YAG (neodymium: yttrium–aluminium–garnet), CO_2 and argon can be appropriate for superficial lesions: CIS, Ta and T1. Although the results are reasonable, it is difficult to assess the depth of penetration. Sensation can be diminished. Biopsies must be taken at any point where a recurrence is thought to have occurred.

Partial penectomy

Preoperative
- Blood tests – haemoglobin
- Urea and electrolytes
- Liver function tests
- Cross-match for 2 units.

Consent
It should be made quite clear that a substantial portion of the penis will be removed.

Surgical aim
The distal penis is removed, with a 2 cm margin proximal to the tumour. The operation is carried out under tourniquet control and the distal urethra is opened out, often with an inlay of penile skin, to try to prevent urethral stenosis.

Total penectomy

Preoperative
As above, plus cross-match 4 units.

Consent
It must be made abundantly clear that the whole penis will be removed and that the patient will need to sit down to pass water. This is the most radical of procedures to be employed. Stenosis of the urethra commonly occurs. Traditionally, the testicles are removed also.

Lymphatic drainage and regional lymph nodes

The urethra and glans penis drain mainly into the superficial lymph nodes, but occasionally into the deep inguinal nodes. The corpora cavernosa drain into the superficial and deep inguinal lymph nodes. Because of free anastomoses of the lymphatic channels, involvement of both sets of nodes is common. It is recommended that the superficial nodes be biopsied. This is known as sentinel node biopsy. The sentinel node is situated at the junction of the saphenous and femoral veins, near the superficial epigastric vein.[6]

Lymph nodes can be assessed by computed tomography (CT) scanning, ultrasound or magnetic resonance imaging (MR) and, where necessary, by fine needle aspiration (FNA).[7] Better results are obtained by immediate lymph node dissection. The lymph nodes should be excised widely, along with overlying subcutaneous tissue. About 50% of patients will be cured by excision of lymph nodes. Many surgeons will wait for 4–6 weeks, placing the patient on antibiotics during this time. Any palpable nodes after this time are an indication for bilateral lymphadenectomy.[8–10]

Neoadjuvant therapy

Cisplatin, bleomycin, methotrexate and 5-fluorouracil (5-FU) have activity in squamous cell carcinomas of the penis.[2] It is claimed that neoadjuvant chemotherapy may make surgery easier, although there are no convincing studies to justify this.

Radiotherapy

Radiotherapy may be used, particularly using small fractions and radiotherapy to the regional lymphatics.

Interstitial therapy produces a uniform dose distribution and can be used for both superficial and deep cancers.[10]

PENILE CANCER CASE HISTORY (patient permission obtained)

A 63-year-old retired fisherman presented to his general practitioner (GP), complaining of a growth in his penis. The GP felt a 2 cm growth and diagnosed this as a penile carcinoma. The patient admitted to only having noticed it in the last few days.

In the past, he has had a myocardial infarction 13 years previously, but is otherwise well.

On closer questioning, it was apparent that he had had a phimosis and had been unable to retract his foreskin for some time.

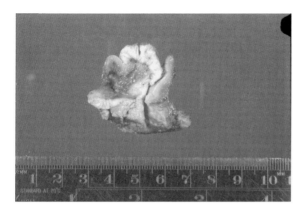

Figure 8.3 Squamous cell cancer of penis protruding through foreskin.

He did not wish anything done initially because he was going on a cruise (!).

He was admitted several days following his cruise and, under examination, it became apparent that the carcinoma was more advanced than was previously thought; i.e. T2, M0, N0. He had no lymphadenopathy, but the carcinoma had pushed its way through the phimosis and it was at that point that he had become aware of it.

A partial penectomy was undertaken.

Histology

A single universal container with three fragments of tissue was received. The first fragment was white, coiled and was of uncertain origin. The second fragment comprised foreskin through which herniated a keratotic white abnormality protruding up to 2.2 cm. This had a dumbbell pattern of growth, with a superficial keratotic expansile head, and a thin stalk. The third fragment comprised mostly white tumour and possibly urethra and substance of the glans.

Histological sections demonstrated a well-differentiated squamous cell carcinoma arising from widespread balanitis xerotica obliterans, albeit with no obvious penile intraepithelial

neoplasia. The diagnosis of a verrucous carcinoma (extremely well-differentiated squamous cell carcinoma) was considered, but focal atypia and irregularity at the base was considered too severe for a verrucous carcinoma diagnosis. The invasive tumour extended into the stroma for approximately 0.7 cm but did not reach the substance of the corpus spongiosum. The squamous-lined urethra was unremarkable, and the painted resection margin was free of invasive disease.

He underwent a CT scan of his pelvis, abdomen and chest, which showed a tiny peripheral lesion in his lungs, but this was thought to be a scar rather than metastasis.

On initial follow-up he was passing his urine well, with no evidence of any recurrence. He will be followed up intensively over the next few months to ensure that there is no local recurrence. We will be paying particular attention to any local recurrence or lymphadenopathy.

Patients who have had a partial penectomy can also develop a stenosis of the urethra. A large flap of penile skin was inlaid into the urethra, to try to prevent this. We would have to be rather guarded about his long-term prognosis.

REFERENCES

1. Masters WH, Johnson VE. Human sexual response. Boston: Little, Brown, 1966
2. Fisher HAG, Perrotti M. Diagnostic evaluation and surgical therapy for penile cancer. In: Testicular and penile cancer, Ernstoff E, Heaney JA, Peschel RE (eds). Oxford: Blackwell Science, 1998
3. Ernstoff E, Heaney JA, Peschel RE (eds). Testicular and penile cancer. Oxford: Blackwell Science, 1998
4. Parkin DM, Whelan SL, Ferlay J, Raymond L, Young J (eds). Cancer incidence in five continents, Vol. VII. IARC Scientific Publications No. 143, Lyon: International Agency for Research on Cancer, 1997
5. Mohs FE, Snow SN, Messing EM, Kuglitsch ME. Microscopically controlled surgery in the treatment of carcinoma of the penis. J Urol 1985; 133:961
6. Horenblas S. Lymphadenectomy for squamous

cell carcinoma of the penis. Part 1: diagnosis of lymph node metastasis. BJU Int 2001; 88:467–472

7. Horenblas S. Lymphadenectomy for squamous cell carcinoma of the penis. Part 2: the role and technique of lymph node dissection. BJU Int 2001; 88:473–483

8. Johnson DE, Lo RK. Complications of groin dissection in penile cancer. Experience with 101 lymphadenectomies. Urology 1984; 24:312–314

9. Horenblas S, Van Tinteren H, Delemarre JFM, Moonen LFM, Lustig V, Van Waardenburg EW. Squamous cell carcinoma of the penis. III Treatment of the regional nodes. J Urol 1993; 149:492–497

10. Pilepich MV. Radiation therapy for penile cancer. In: Testicular and penile cancer, Ernstoff E, Heaney JA, Peschel RE (eds). Oxford: Blackwell Science, 1998

9

Urethral cancer

INCIDENCE

- Male : female – 1 : 4
- <1% genitourinary cancers in men
- <0.02% genitourinary cancers in women.[2]

PATHOLOGY

Squamous cell carcinoma represents 75% of all urethral cancers in women and about 50% of urethral cancers in men.

Transitional cell carcinomas represent 15% of cancers in both sexes and adenocarcinomas represent 15% of tumours in women and 5% in men.[2,3]

AETIOLOGY

- Largely unknown
- In men, a sizeable proportion have had urethral stricture, and up to one-half have had venereal disease.

STAGING

The TNM (tumour, node, metastasis) staging system for urethral tumours is shown in Table 9.1.

SURVIVAL

Females

- Radiotherapy: 34% at 5 years
- Surgery + radiotherapy: 55% at 5 years.

Table 9.1 Summary of TNM staging of urethral tumours in female and male	
Stage	**Finding**
Tx	Primary tumour cannot be assessed
T0	No evidence of primary tumour
Ta	Non-invasive papillary, polypoid or verrucous
Tis	In situ
T1	Invading subepithelial connective tissue
T2	Invading corpus spongiosum, prostate or periurethral muscle
T3	Invading corpus cavernosum, anterior vagina or beyond bladder neck or prostatic capsule
T4	Invading other adjacent organs
N1	Single <2 cm
N2	>2 cm (but <5 cm) or multiple
N3	Lymph node metastasis >5 cm in greatest dimension

Males

Survival is 20% at 5 years.

DIAGNOSIS

- An examination under anaesthesia (EUA) and cystoscopy allow biopsies to be taken
- In the female, the urethra is generally indurated.

STAGING INVESTIGATIONS

- Chest X-ray
- Bone scan
- CT (computed tomography) scan.[4]

TREATMENT

Females

Local surgical excision or laser excision may be adequate. The risk is of post-therapy incontinence, but generally it is better to sacrifice this to obtain adequate margins.[5,6]

Radiotherapy can be curative with more advanced local disease, or can allow local palliation.[7]

Males

Because this condition is so rare, there are few series and fewer trials. Carcinoma of the distal urethra can be treated by partial penectomy, with a 2 cm margin of tissue free from tumour.

For more aggressive tumours, treatment may require en bloc resection of the penis.[8–10]

Chemotherapy and chemo/radiotherapy

Most of these techniques have been tried in an attempt at penis preservation. Limited success has been reported, but most attempts are limited by the radiosensitivity of the perineum.[11–13]

PROGNOSTIC FACTORS

Anterior position (presumably because they present earlier).

URETHRAL CANCER IN A FEMALE PATIENT CASE HISTORY

An 81-year-old lady presented via her family practitioner, with severe left iliac fossa and left loin pain and urinary symptoms. She was admitted under the care of the gynaecologists, who found her to have a bulky uterus and a hard nodule on the cervix and also a hard nodule on anterior portion of the urethra; both of these were biopsied.

The patient had a past history of non-Hodgkin's lymphoma.

A CT scan was non-contributory.

The biopsies indicated poorly differentiated adenocarcinoma. Despite the biopsies, there was some doubt as to the site of the primary, but it was eventually concluded that it was urethra, T2. She had a palliative course of external beam radiotherapy, 20 Gy in four fractions.

Her treatment was complicated with diverticulitis and a urinary tract infection.

She was unable to void spontaneously and required a long-term catheter. She was unable to mobilise and later in the month, about 3 weeks after the start of her treatment, she suffered a major intracerebral event. Her condition deteriorated rapidly and she died peacefully the following day, with her relatives present.

Comment

This is a fairly typical case of the rare number of patients who present with primary urethral tumours. The diagnosis can often be in doubt and, initially, it was suspected that she was suffering from a further manifestation of her non-Hodgkins's lymphoma.

She made a poor response to radiotherapy treatment but, as is often the case, died from other causes, which were probably unrelated.

REFERENCES

1. Shakespeare W. Hamlet I iv 32. The Alexander Edition of William Shakespeare. The Complete Works. London: Collins, 1951.
2. Terry P, Cookson MS, Sarosdy MF. Carcinoma of the urethra and scrotum. In: Principles and practice of genitourinary oncology, Raghavan D, Scher HI, Leibel SA, Lange P (eds). Philadelphia: Lippincott-Raven, 1997
3. Mostofi FK, Davis CJ Jr, Sesterhenn IA. Cancer of male and female urethra. Urol Clin North Am 1992; 19:347–358
4. Vapnek JM, Hricak H, Carroll PR. Recent advances in imaging studies for staging penile and urethral cancer. Urol Clin North Am 1992; 19:259–266
5. Narayan P, Korety B. Surgical techniques of female urethral cancer. Urol Clin North Am 1992; 19:373–382
6. Moinuddin Ali M, Klein FA, Hazra TA. Primary female urethral carcinoma: a retrospective comparison of different treatment techniques. Cancer 1988; 62:54–57
7. Forman JD, Lichter AS. The role of radiation therapy in the management of carcinoma of the male and female urethra. Urol Clin North Am 1992; 19:383–389
8. Marshall VF. Radical excision of locally extensive carcinoma of the deep male urethra. J Urol 1957; 78:252–264
9. Ray B, Canto SR, Whitmore WF Jr. Experience with primary carcinoma of the male urethra. J Urol 1977; 117:591–594
10. Zeidman EJ, Desmond P, Thompson IM. Surgical techniques of carcinoma of the male urethra. Urol Clin North Am 1992; 19:359–372
11. Baskin LS, Tuzan C. Carcinoma of male urethra, management of locally advanced disease with combined chemo/radiotherapy and penile preserving surgery. Urology 1992; 39:21–25
12. Hussein AM, Benedetto P, Sridhar KS. Chemotherapy with cisplatin and 5-fluorouracil for penile and urethral squamous cell carcinomas. Cancer 1990; 65:433–438
13. Johnson DW, Kessler JF, Ferrigni RG. Low-dose combined chemo/radiotherapy in the management of locally advanced urethral squamous cell carcinoma. J Urol 1989; 141:615–616

FURTHER READING

Levine RL. Urethral cancer. Cancer 1980; 45(7 suppl):1965–1972.

10

The interface between urology and gynaecological cancer

Were it in my choice, I would reject a petrarchal coronation – on account of my dying day, and because women have cancers

John Keats[1]

It is unnecessary to go into great detail about gynaecological cancer. The urologist will be asked to come and deal with patients who are already under the care of a specialist and an oncologist who will have a much deeper involvement with advanced disease than is appropriate for this particular book.

The following notes are, however, included to give a working knowledge of the important gynaecological cancers.

CANCER OF THE CERVIX

INCIDENCE

Cervical cancer is second only to breast cancer in worldwide incidence. There is wide variation in incidence and lifetime risk: England and Wales is 1.25%, whereas it is only 0.5% in Israel. This may be due to males being circumcised, but there may be other factors, such as poverty, which may be involved.[2]

PRE-INVASIVE DISEASE OF THE CERVIX

Almost all cancers of the cervix can be detected at an early stage by cervical screening. These programmes are credited with an overall drop in incidence of the disease, despite the fact that the disease is more prevalent. The disease presents in an early stage, between the ages of 25 and 40, but invasive disease peaks between 35 and 50.[2]

CAUSES

It is thought that the number of sexual partners and the age at first intercourse are important. There is believed also to be a risk associated with the woman's partner, where he has had multiple sexual partners. The incidence is reduced when barrier contraception is used, but is increased in women who smoke, which appears to affect the immunity of the cervix.

It is thought that transmissible agents play a strong role in the development of the cancer. The two agents most commonly discussed by us are the herpes simplex virus 2 (HSV2), but more popularly now, human papillomaviruses (HPV).[2]

The spread of the disease

Cervical carcinoma spreads by direct invasion and by lymphatics. Direct spread involves spread into the body of the uterus and into the vaginal mucosa. The ligaments of the uterus and pelvic side wall may become involved and it is at this stage that the ureters can be constricted. Very occasionally the bladder can be invaded anteriorly and the rectum posteriorly.

Distant spread is unusual and many women

will die with local disease only. Metastases occasionally occur to the lungs, bone and liver.[2]

PATHOLOGY

Nine out of ten of invasive cervical carcinomas are squamous carcinomas.

SYMPTOMS

The commonest symptom is that of postcoital, intermenstrual or postmenopausal bleeding. Vaginal discharge is the second commonest symptom. Pain occurs in advanced cases with direct muscle or nerve involvement. Rectal bleeding and haematuria can be symptoms of advanced disease.[2]

TREATMENT OF INVASIVE DISEASE

Surgery is the best treatment for younger patients, with small volume disease. Treatment involves radical hysterectomy and pelvic lymphadenectomy. This is often termed 'Wertheim's' hysterectomy. The vaginal epithelium is removed as a cuff in this procedure. The ovaries are usually preserved.[2]

RADIOTHERAPY

This is reserved for older women or more bulky tumours. It can result in fibrosis and damage to the vaginal size and flexibility.[2]

COMPLICATIONS OF SURGERY

Bladder injury

Bladder drainage may be compromised and the patient may have to start self-catheterisation. There is a risk of fistula formation, involving the ureters or small bowel. This problem is worse after surgery for recurrence after radical radiotherapy. Lymphadenectomy can lead to

lymph collections, which can of themselves obstruct the ureters.[3]

Ureteric fistulae

The major complication of radical hysterectomy is that of ureteric fistula. This seems to be more common after radiotherapy and this may be due to damage to the blood supply to the ureter. The ureter is more liable to necrosis and fistulas then form subsequently.

One useful tip where the pelvic dissection is anticipated to be technically difficult, is to insert bilateral ureteric catheters before opening the abdomen. These make ureteric identification much easier and the catheters can be withdrawn at the end of the procedure.[4]

Surgery plus radiotherapy

If surgery is followed by radiotherapy, the complications tend to increase; these complications may be dose-related. Various rates of fistula after surgery alone have been noted, ranging from 0 to 4.8%. The rates of vesical damage are lower and range from 0 to 4.2%.

Radiotherapy alone

The complications after radiotherapy alone are those of vesicovaginal fistula, radiation ulcers, a shrunken bladder and haemorrhagic cystitis.[5,6] Ureteric injury following radiotherapy has been described.[7]

SURGERY TO REPAIR FISTULA

This is a topic which would require a book on its own. The most popular method of repair is that of the omental-pedicle graft, as popularised by Turner-Warwick. The fistula is exposed, usually from above, and the deficiency repaired in two layers. The greater omentum is dissected and a tail with a good supply is prepared. This is then overlaid on the repair and sutured in position. The omentum introduces a new blood supply to the area; the success rate is very high.[8]

COMPLICATIONS OF RADIOTHERAPY FOR GYNAECOLOGICAL CANCERS

These complications include radiation cystitis; late effects are normally bowel-related, and may be absorption of bowel salts, leading to diarrhoea, or vitamin B_{12}. The ureters can be constricted, leading to hydronephrosis. If this occurs however, it is always sensible to rule out tumour recurrence, which is regrettably more common.

CHEMOTHERAPY

Drugs commonly in use are cisplatin, methotrexate and ifosfamide: these drugs are all potentially nephrotoxic and glomerular filtration rates should be estimated. The side effects of these drugs require to be monitored:[2]

Cisplatin
Peripheral neuropathy
High tone hearing loss
Tinnitus

Methotrexate
Myelosuppression
Folinic acid can be used as a 'rescue'

Ifosfamide
Central nervous system problems, i.e. hallucinations and irritability

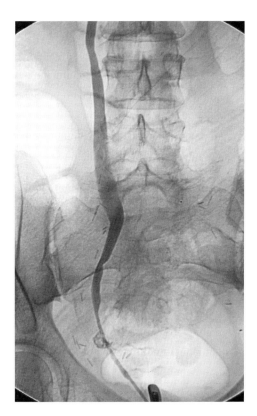

Figure 10.1 Right retrograde pyelogram in a patient 3 weeks post radical hysterectomy demonstrating contrast leakage from distal right ureter. The patient was leaking *per vaginam*.

CASE HISTORY (patient permission obtained)

A 38-year-old lady was seen at a colposcopy clinic because her cervical smear showed glandular abnormalities. A cervical biopsy was performed and this revealed nuclear hyperchromasia and nuclear enlargement, consistent with moderate atypia (CGIN). She was therefore admitted for hysteroscopy, fractional curettage and cone biopsy under general anaesthetic.

The cone biopsy revealed that she had adenocarcinoma. This was measured at 1.6 cm × 1.0 cm × 1.2 cm, with lymphatic space invasion, and was not completely excised. It was diagnosed as at least a stage 1B adenocarcinoma of the cervix. She was a para 2 + 0 and she was happy to proceed to a hysterectomy for health reasons.

She was therefore admitted for a radical abdominal hysterectomy and pelvic lymph node dissection. Her ovaries were not removed. The operation appeared to be uneventful. The patient's catheter was removed on the 14th postoperative day. She subsequently complained of a watery discharge. A swab test was undertaken with blue dye but was negative and she seemed to be passing urine normally.

However, the comment was made that she continued to pass frequent small amounts of urine and continued to have urinary incontinence, with frequent pad changes.

An intravenous urogram (IVU) was requested by the urologists who were consulted and moderate hydronephrosis was seen. She was transferred to the Urology Department and had a cystoscopy and right retrograde pyelogram. Cystoscopy revealed bullous oedema on the right side of the bladder.

The retrograde pyelogram showed a ureteric stricture at the lower end of the right ureter with escape of contrast into the vagina. Because the lady lived a great distance from the hospital, we elected to attempt an insertion of a right ureteric stent, following the demonstration of the ureteric fistula in the right ureter. A Terumo wire was used to cross the stricture in the lower pelvic ureter and there was a moderate hydronephrosis. A 6F 22 cm stent was inserted successfully. The leak was once again demonstrated as just above the vesicoureteric junction.

When the stent was removed 3 months later, there was still a small leak *per vaginam*. A decision was made to carry out a laparotomy and the fistula was identified. This was closed in two layers, allowing the stent to remain *in situ*. The whole area was then vascularised, using a pedicle of omentum.

The lady made a quick complete recovery from this and her stent was removed 2 weeks after her laparotomy.

Comment

The mechanism of ureteric injury is not always direct trauma, but may be caused by ischaemia. Nonetheless, an index of suspicion is necessary, despite a negative pad test, with a patient with these symptoms.

> It is recommended that transfer to the Urology Department be undertaken at an early stage.

REFERENCES

1. Keats J. Letters, 66, to Benjamin Bailey, 10th June 1818
2. Blake P. Cervix in treatment of cancer, 3rd edn, Price P, Sikora K (eds). London: Chapman & Hall Medical, 1995
3. Parkin DE, Davis JA, Symonds RP. Urodynamic findings following radiotherapy for cervical carcinoma. Br J Urol 1988; 61:213–217
4. Parkin DE. Lower urinary tract complications of the treatment of cervical carcinoma. Obstet Gynaecol Surv 1989; 44(7):523–529
5. Kunz J. Urological complications in gynaecological surgery and radiotherapy. Contrib Gynaecol Obstet 1984; 11:1 5
6. Jones CR, Woodhouse CRJ, Hendry WF. Urological problems following treatment of carcinoma of the cervix. Br J Urol 1984; 56:609–613
7. Underwood PB, Lutz MH, Smoak LM. Ureteral injury following irradiation therapy for carcinoma of the cervix. Obstet Gynaecol 1977; 49: 663–667
8. Turner-Warwick RT. The use of the omental pedicle graft in urinary tract reconstruction. J Urol 1976; 116:341–347

11

Palliative care and pain control

[Physicians] should not allow [the patient] to be tormented with useless and annoying applications, in a disease of settled destiny. It should be remembered that all cases are susceptible of errors of commission as well as omission, and that by an excessive application of means of art, we may frustrate the intentions of nature, when they are salutary, or embitter the approach of death when it is inevitable.

Jacob Bigelow[1]

He has seen but half the universe who has not been shown the house of pain.

Ralph Waldo Emerson[2]

GENERAL COMMENTARY

There comes a point unfortunately on the patient journey where your best efforts have proved fruitless. Sometimes, the patient may feel completely well: e.g. a patient with a rising prostate-specific antigen (PSA) has failed both primary and secondary hormonal manipulations. If a patient is functioning well, both you and the patient may realise that although things are satisfactory at present, it will eventually catch up with the patient. You may have made this point at an earlier stage, discussing the disease with the patient, to say that you may well be able to control it for quite some time but that it will eventually return.

It is part of the art of medicine to know at what stage in the patient's illness to introduce the concept of palliative care. To some extent, this is part of every doctor's duty throughout the management of a patient with a terminal condition, but it is recognised that physicians who specialise in palliative care have a greater expertise to offer.

The World Health Organization defines palliative care as

the act of total care of patients whose disease is not responsive to curative treatment. Control of pain, of other symptoms and of psychological, social and spiritual problems is paramount. The goal of palliative care is the achievement of the best possible quality of life for a patient and their families.[3]

It is often difficult for a specialist to accept that the best endeavour of the physician is not to cure or to prolong life but to increase the quality of the remaining life left. It is important to maintain contact with the patient to assess their problems.

PAIN

- The presence of new continued pain affects over 50% of cancer patients and this increases to 75% in the terminal stages
- There is an escalation of drugs used to control pain, and this proceeds from simple analgesics through to opioids
- This is illustrated in the WHO analgesic ladder.[3]

QUICK REFERENCE SUMMARY (with grateful acknowledgement to the Scottish Intercollegiate Guidelines Network[4])

Principles of management of pain in patients with cancer

These short points are a guide to pain control for most non-experts:

Patients should be given information and instruction about pain and pain management and be encouraged to take an active role in their pain management.

The principles of treatment outlined in the WHO Cancer Pain Relief programme should be followed when treating pain in patients with cancer.

For appropriate use of the WHO analgesic ladder, analgesics should be selected depending upon initial assessment and the dose titrated as a result of ongoing regular reassessment of response.

A patient's treatment should start at the step of the WHO analgesic ladder appropriate for the severity of the pain.

If the pain severity increases and is not controlled on a given step, move upwards to the next step of the analgesic ladder. Do not prescribe another analgesic of the same potency.

All patients with moderate to severe cancer pain, regardless of aetiology, should receive a trial of opioid analgesia.

Analgesia for continuous pain should be prescribed on a regular basis, not 'as required'.

Education

One of the keys to pain control is education for health care staff.

Pre-registration curricula for health care professionals should place greater emphasis on pain management education

Continuing pain management education programmes should be available to all health care professionals caring for patients with cancer.

Assessment

Accurate assessment of the patient is essential.

Prior to treatment an accurate assessment should be performed to determine the type (Box 11.1) and severity of pain, and its effect on the patient

The patient should be the prime assessor of his or her pain

For effective pain control the physical, functional, psychosocial and spiritual dimensions should be assessed

A simple formal assessment tool should be used in the ongoing assessment of pain

All health care professionals involved in cancer care should be educated and trained in assessing pain as well as in the principles of its control

Sudden severe pain should be recognised as a medical emergency and patients should be seen and assessed without delay.

Box 11.1   Types of pain

Somatic
Visceral
Neuropathic
Sympathetically mediated
Mixed
Anguish

Psychosocial issues

A thorough assessment of the patient's psychological and social state should be carried out. This should include assessment of anxiety and, in particular, depression, as well as the patient's beliefs about pain.

CHOICE OF ANALGESIA FOR CANCER PAIN

The WHO analgesic ladder

Step 1: Mild pain
Non-opioids ± adjuvant (Box 11.4).

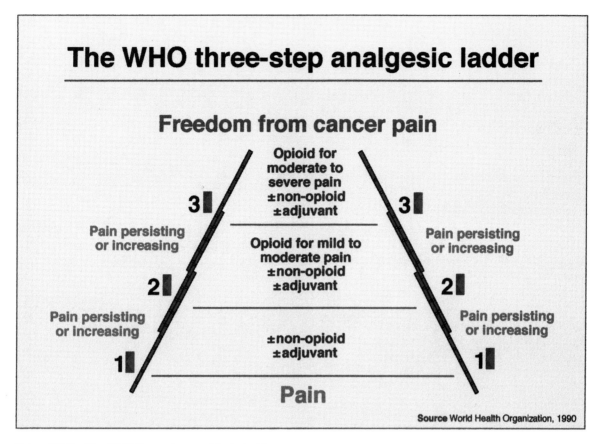

Figure 11.1 The WHO three-step analgesic ladder.

<table>
</table>

Box 11.2 Freedom from cancer pain: drug options	
First line Morphine Diamorphine + step 1 non-opioids	Morphine or diamorphine should be used to treat moderate to severe pain in patients with cancer
Alternative Fentanyl Hydromorphone Methadone Oxycodone Phenazocine + step 1 non-opioids	The oral route is the recommended route of administration and should be used where possible A trial of alternative opioids should be considered for moderate to severe pain where dose titration is limited by side effects of morphine or diamorphine

Step 2: Mild to moderate pain
Opioid for mild to moderate pain plus a non-opioid ± adjuvant (Box 11.3).

Step 3: Moderate to severe pain
Opioid for moderate to severe pain plus a non-opioid ± adjuvant (Box 11.2).

Use of opioids in treatment of moderate to severe cancer pain

Initiating and titrating oral morphine
   When initiating normal-release morphine, start with 5–10 mg orally at 4-hourly intervals, unless there are contraindications
   The opioid dose for each patient should be titrated to achieve maximum analgesia and minimum side effects for that patient

---

Box 11.3   Pain persisting or increasing: drug options

Codeine Dihydrocodeine Dextropropoxyphene + step 1 non- opioids	Patients with mild to moderate pain should receive codeine, dihydrocodeine or dextropropoxyphene plus paracetamol or a nonsteroidal anti-inflammatory drug (NSAID)
	If the effect of an opioid for mild to moderate pain at optimum dose is not adequate, do not change to another opioid for mild to moderate pain. Move to step 3 of the analgesic ladder
	Compound analgesics containing subtherapeutic doses of opioids for mild to moderate pain should not be used for pain control in patients with cancer

---

Box 11.4   Pain persisting or increasing: drug options

Paracetamol Aspirin Nonsteroidal anti-inflammatory drugs (NSAIDs)	Patients with mild pain should receive either an NSAID or paracetamol at licensed doses. The choice should be based on a risk/benefit analysis for each individual patient
	Patients receiving an NSAID who are at risk of gastrointestinal side effects* should be prescribed misoprostol (200 µg, two or three times a day) or omeprazole (20 mg, once a day)

*Includes patients aged >60 years, smokers, those with previous peptic ulcer, those on steroids or anticoagulants and patients with existing renal or hepatic disease or cardiac failure.

Where possible, titration should be carried out with a normal-release morphine preparation

Once suitable pain control is achieved by the use of normal-release morphine, conversion to the same total daily dose of controlled-release morphine should be considered.

Breakthrough analgesia

Every patient on opioids for moderate to severe pain should have access to breakthrough analgesia, usually in the form of normal-release morphine.

Breakthrough analgesia should be one-sixth of the total regular daily dose of oral morphine.

Following the delivery of oral breakthrough analgesia, wait 30 min to assess the response. If pain persists, repeat analgesia and reassess in a further 30 min. If pain still persists, full reassessment of the patient is required.

Careful explanation of the correct use of breakthrough analgesia to carers and patients is necessary.

Predictable side effects

Constipation: patients receiving an opioid must have access to regular prophylactic laxatives. A combination of stimulant and softening laxative will be required.

Nausea and vomiting: patients commencing an opioid for moderate to severe pain should have access to a prophylactic antiemetic to be taken if required.

Sedation: patients receiving opioids for moderate to severe pain for the first time should be warned that sedation may occur and be advised of the risks of driving or using machinery. The use of other sedative drugs or drugs with sedative side effects should be rationalised.

Dry mouth: all patients should be educated on the need for, and methods of achieving, good oral hygiene.

Alternative opioids can be tried in patients with opioid-sensitive pain who are unable to tolerate morphine side effects.

Opioid toxicity, tolerance and dependence

Opioid toxicity should be managed by reducing the dose of opioid, ensuring adequate hydration and treating the agitation/confusion with haloperidol (1.5–3 mg, orally or subcutaneously). This dose can be repeated hourly in the acute situation.

Initiation of opioid analgesia should not be delayed by anxiety over pharmacological tolerance, as in clinical practice this does not occur.

Initiation of opioids should not be delayed due to unfounded fears concerning psychological dependence.

Patients should be reassured that they will not become psychologically dependent on their opioid analgesia.

Parenteral administration

Patients requiring parenteral opioids should receive the appropriate dose of diamorphine via the subcutaneous route.

To calculate the 24-hour dose of subcutaneous diamorphine, divide the total 24-hour oral dose of morphine by 3. Administer this dose of diamorphine subcutaneously over 24 hours.

Safe systems for use and management of syringe drivers must be in place as detailed in guidance issued by the Scottish Department of Health.

Adjuvant analgesics

Patients with neuropathic pain should have a trial of a tricyclic antidepressant and/or an anticonvulsant.

A therapeutic trial or oral high-dose dexamethasone should be considered for raised intracranial pressure, severe bone pain, nerve infiltration or compression, pressure due to soft tissue swelling or infiltration, spinal cord compression or hepatic capsular pain (unless there are contraindications). In some clinical situations (e.g. if the patient is vomiting) it may be necessary to use the intravenous route.

Mexiletine should not be used routinely as an adjuvant analgesic. Details of some adjuvant analgesics are given in Table 11.1.

SUMMARY OF RECOMMENDATIONS: ASSESSMENT OF PAIN IN PATIENTS WITH CANCER

Prior to treatment an accurate assessment should be performed to determine the type and severity of pain, and its effect on the patient

The patient should be the prime assessor of his or her pain

For effective pain control, the physical, functional, psychosocial and spiritual dimensions should be assessed

The severity of pain and the overall distress caused to the patient should be differentiated and each treated appropriately

A simple formal assessment tool should be used in the ongoing assessment of pain

All health care professionals involved in cancer care should be educated and trained in assessing pain as well as in the principles of its control

Sudden severe pain in patients with cancer should be recognised by all health professionals as a medical emergency and patients should be seen and assessed without delay.

DEFINITIONS OF PAIN

Pain has been defined in many ways:

- 'An unpleasant sensory and emotional experience associated with actual or potential tissue damage, or described in terms of such damage'[5]
- 'Pain is a category of complex experiences, not a single sensation produced by a single stimulus'[5]
- 'Pain is what the experiencing person says it is, existing whenever he says it does'[5]

Table 11.1 Some adjuvant analgesics			
Drug	**Dosage**	**Indications**	**Main side effects**
Nonsteroidal anti-inflammatory drugs (NSAIDS): e.g. ibuprofen, diclofenac	400–600 mg qid 50 mg po tds (sr 75 mg bd) 100 mg pr daily	Bone metastases Soft tissue infiltration Liver pain	Gastric irritation Gastric bleeding Fluid retention Headache Vertigo Renal impairment
Steroids: e.g. dexamethasone	8–16 mg/day	Raised intracranial pressure Nerve compression Soft tissue infiltration Liver pain Bone pain	Gastric irritation if together with NSAID Fluid retention Confusion/agitation Cushingoid appearance Carbohydrate intolerance Oral candidiasis
Tricyclic antidepressants: e.g. amitriptyline	25 mg nocte (starting dose) median effective dose: 75 mg nocte	Neuropathic pain	Sedation Dizziness Postural hypotension Dry mouth Constipation Urinary retention
Anticonvulsants: e.g. carbamazepine	200 mg nocte (starting dose) rising to 1600 mg	Nerve pain	Vertigo Nausea Constipation Rash

sr = slow release, pr = per rectum.

BACKGROUND

Many patients think cancer and pain are synonymous, but the reality is more complex:

- one-third of patients with cancer do not experience severe pain
- of the two-thirds of cancer patients who do experience severe pain, around 88% can and should have their pain adequately controlled by the application of basic principles of pain management[5]
- of those cancer patients who have pain, 80% have more than two pains and 40% have pain before the terminal phase of their illness.[5]

Specialists who may be able to assist with patients who have difficult pain problems include palliative care physicians, clinical nurse specialists (CNS), pain relief anaesthetists, pharmacists, psychologists, occupational therapists and physiotherapists.

The patient should be the prime assessor of his or her pain.

ASSESSMENT OF PAIN

1. Physical effects/manifestations of pain[5]
2. Functional effects – interference with activities of daily living[5]
3. Psychosocial factors – level of anxiety, mood, cultural influences, fears, effects on interpersonal relationships, factors affecting pain thresholds (Table 11.2).

Kaye[5] details a wide variety of emotions displayed in spiritual pain, and has categorised them in terms of:

- the past (painful memories, regret, failure, guilt)
- the present (isolation, unfairness, anger)
- the future (fear, hopelessness).

History

Detailed history taking is vital to comprehensive assessment. Listen to the patient carefully and determine:

- site and number of pains
- intensity/severity of pains
- radiation of pain
- timing of pain
- quality of pain
- aggravating and relieving factors
- aetiology of pain:
    pain caused by cancer
    pain cause by treatment
    pain associated with cancer-related debility (e.g. decubitus ulcers)
    pain unrelated to cancer or treatment
- type of pain:
    somatic
    visceral
    neuropathic
    sympathetically mediated
    mixed
    anguish
- analgesic drug history
- presence of clinically significant psychological disorder, e.g. anxiety and/or depression.

Physical examination

Ideally, a full physical examination should be undertaken, aimed at reaching a diagnosis and establishing the best effective treatment. If the patient is very weak, an examination targeted to the area of pain may be sufficient.

Table 11.2 Factors affecting pain tolerance	
Aspects that lower pain tolerance	**Aspects that raise pain tolerance**
• Discomfort	• Relief of symptoms
• Insomnia	• Sleep
• Fatigue	• Rest or (paradoxically) physiotherapy
• Anxiety	• Relaxation therapy
• Fear	• Explanation/support
• Anger	• Understanding/empathy
• Boredom	• Diversional activity
• Sadness	• Companionship/listening
• Depression	• Elevation of mood
• Introversion	• Understanding of the meaning and significance of the pain
• Social abandonment	
• Mental isolation	

PHYSICAL AND PSYCHOLOGICAL DEPENDENCE

Psychological dependence on opioids (addiction) generally does not occur in cancer patients experiencing pain:[6]

> initiation of opioids should not be delayed due to unfounded fears concerning psychological dependence
>
> patients should be reassured that they will not become psychologically dependent on their opioid analgesia.

MANAGEMENT OF POSTOPERATIVE PAIN IN PATIENTS ALREADY ON OPIOIDS

> Patients taking opioids preoperatively should be managed in a high-dependency unit postoperatively.

INTERVENTIONAL TECHNIQUES FOR THE TREATMENT OF PAIN FROM CANCER

Interventional techniques to relieve pain in patients with cancer should only be considered in the following circumstances:

1. Standard treatments such as systemic drug therapy (oral, transdermal, subcutaneous, etc.) have been tried and failed. Failure may be due to insufficient pain relief or unacceptable side effects.
2. Personal, psychological and social circumstances should have been evaluated.
3. Other causes for incomplete analgesia should have been excluded.
4. The patient should be fit enough for the procedure.
5. The patient must be able to give informed consent.
6. The patient's pain must be likely to respond to the procedure.

Epidural and intrathecal drug delivery systems may be considered. Cordotomy is occasionally effective as a last resort.

> All professionals looking after patients with pain from cancer should be aware of the range of neurosurgical and anaesthetic techniques available for the relief of pain
>
> All professionals looking after patients with pain from cancer should have access to a specialist pain relief service that is able to offer the techniques described above
>
> If a patient's pain is not controlled by other measures, then the advice of a specialist in pain relief should be sought, with a view to performing one of the above procedures
>
> After successful interventional procedures patients already on opioids should have the dose reduced by approximately one-third
>
> After interventional procedures, patients on opioids should be carefully supervised for increased signs of opioid toxicity.

KEY MESSAGES FOR PATIENTS

- Not all patients with cancer have pain.
- Patients with cancer who do experience pain should not accept uncontrolled pain as part of their condition.
- Most pain can be well controlled. In difficult cases, the pain can at least be reduced in severity.
- A patient with cancer can experience pain due to non-cancer-related illness.
- Increasing pain does not mean death is imminent.
- Patients and their carers should have a full explanation of how to take their medication, including the indications for the drug, the name of the drug, how often to take it, how to deal with breakthrough and incident pain and the possible side effects of the drug.
- Patients with chronic pain should be prescribed regular analgesics with analgesic strength commensurate to the level of pain.
- Analgesics invariably produce constipation, and prescribed laxatives should be taken as instructed.
- Patients should be informed of the availability of appropriate clinical trials. When this information is provided it should also be stated that there is no obligation for patients to participate in any trial.

- Barriers to the use of opioids for pain control are fear of tolerance or addiction. Starting morphine or another opioid early does not mean the dose will steadily increase to a very large dose and that if pain increases there will be no suitable analgesic available. Patients with cancer who have pain and are prescribed morphine-type analgesic do not develop psychological dependency. Being commenced on opioids does not mean death is imminent.
- A patient who is unhappy with his level of pain control has the right to ask to be referred to a palliative medicine physician or anaesthetist specialising in pain control. Requesting this will not affect how he is treated by his present physician.

CONTROL OF NAUSEA AND VOMITING

If possible, identify the cause of the nausea or vomiting. If it is due to delayed gastric emptying, it may be that a drug such as Maxolon (metoclopramide) may be effective. Opioid therapy produces reduction in the gastrointestinal tract activity, as well as having central effects on vomiting.

It is important to seek the help of experienced personnel rather than trying to soldier on unaided.

Dopamine antagonists such as haloperidol or Prophloresine act centrally.

Corticosteroids can reduce intracranial pressure and reduce vomiting and may also have a role where there is a large burden of hepatic metastases.

CONTROL OF CONSTIPATION

Poor intake and opioid therapy reduce constipation. Faecal impaction may occur, and this responds to local measures such as enemata or disimpaction. Regular use of suppositories may prevent this from happening. The help of experienced practitioners should be sought at an early stage where constipation is a problem and this is best dealt with by a team approach.

10 KEY POINTS FOR CANCER CARE

1. Recognise the person with cancer as someone with rights, opinions and a possible desire to be involved in their own care.
2. Provide information at the point of diagnosis with reference to the cancer, treatment, options and prognosis. This information should be given with clear explanations at an appropriate time and in an appropriate place.
3. Provide information about support groups and other sources of help.
4. Make available counselling support both to the patient, the family and/or carers, including any children.
5. Make available counselling support at all stages, including bereavement counselling.
6. Provide a focal point at localised centres, which offer information and support helping to relieve the sense of isolation.
7. Ensure better communication between hospital and primary care medical/nursing services.
8. Initiate further training for community medical/nursing staff in palliative care.
9. Ensure speedier access to services like Macmillan nurses.
10. Make available a 'named' key worker/carer.

REFERENCES

1. Bigelow J. Nature in disease. Boston: Ticknor and Fields, 1854 [as cited in Rushton AR. Genetics and medicine in the United States, p 18]
2. Emerson RW. Society and solitude, 1870. Republished: Boston: Houghton, Mifflin, 1904
3. World Health Organization. Technical Report CA 804, Cancer, pain and palliative care. Geneva: World Health Organization, 1990
4. Scottish Intercollegiate Guidelines Network, Scottish cancer therapy network. Control of Pain in Patients with Cancer, June 2000
5. Kaye P. Symptom control in hospice and palliative care. Essex, Connecticut: Hospice Education Institute, 1990
6. Fallon MT, de Williams AC, Hanks GW, Ghodse H. Why don't patients with pain become addicted to morphine? Abstract 8th World Congress on Pain, IASP, 1997: 390

FURTHER READING

Classification of chronic pain. Descriptions of chronic pain syndromes and definitions of pain terms. Prepared by the International Association for the Study of Pain, Subcommittee on Taxonomy. Pain 1986; S3:1–226

Cleeland CS, Gonin R, Hatfield AK, et al. Pain and its treatment in outpatients with metastatic cancer. N Engl J Med 1994; 330:592–596

Cleeland CS, Nakamura Y, Mendoza TR, Edwards KR, Douglas J, Serlin RC. Dimensions of the impact of cancer pain in a four country sample: new information from multidimensional scaling. Pain 1996; 67:267–273

Doyle D, Hanks GWC, MacDonald N. Oxford textbook of palliative medicine. Oxford: Oxford University Press, 1993

Faull C. Symptom control in terminal illness. Prescribers J 1998; 38(1):32–39

Lee M, Tiernan E, Chambers WA. The management of pain in urological malignancies. UroOncology 2001; 1:153–160

McCaffery M. Nursing management of the patient in pain. Philadelphia: JB Lippincott, 1972

Melzack R, Wall PD. The challenge of pain. Harmondsworth: Penguin, 1982

O'Boyle CA, Moriarty MJ, Hillard N. Clinical and psychological aspects of cancer-related pain. Ir Psychol Med 1988; 5:89–92

Serlin RC, Mendoza TR, Nakamura Y, Edwards KR, Cleeland CS. When is cancer pain mild, moderate or severe? Grading pain severity by its interference with function. Pain 1995; 61:277–284

Tiernan E. Palliative care in urological cancer. UroOncology 2000; 1:7–10

Twycross R, Lack SA. Symptom control in advanced cancer. London: Pitman Books, 1984

Twycross R, Harcourt J, Bergl S. A survey of pain in patients with advanced cancer. J Pain Sympt Man 1996; 12:273–282

Zech DF, Grond S, Lynch J, Hertel D, Lehmann KA. Validation of World Health Organization guidelines for cancer pain relief a 10 year prospective study. Pain 1995; 63:65–76

12

Communication and bad news

A cancer is not only a physical disease, it is a state of mind

Michael Baden[1]

Formerly, when religion was strong and science weak men mistook magic for medicine; now when science is strong and religion weak men mistake medicine for magic

Thomas Szasz[2]

GENERAL COMMENTARY

It would be expected that students who are attracted into a medical career are 'people persons'; in other words, they enjoy the company of other people and have developed their interpersonal skills to a high level.

This can be true in many instances, but the sad fact is that many of us are not good with people. Perhaps our innate abilities of communication have been squeezed out by educational systems or perhaps, for some, the attraction of the science involved in medicine led to good examination grades and into medical school.

Medical School selectors are aware of this problem and many try to interview students, to exclude social misfits.

Changes in society have meant that the cause of patients has been championed not only as patients but also as consumers, with a right to criticise and complain. In some health systems, this is putting increasing pressure on doctors in situations where their clinics may be busy. This can also be an excuse to cut down patient contact to a minimum, but for patients with cancer,

this is not acceptable. Some consultations with patients may be critical, particularly where bad news or an adverse diagnosis has to be conveyed. I am sure that most readers will accept that patients have a right to this information. It is no longer acceptable to form a conclave with relatives and exclude the patient from information, although this was arguably appropriate in a very paternalistic system previously.

You, as the patient's doctor, have a contract with the patient. That unspoken contract means it is your duty to impart information with honesty and compassion. The touchstone must always be how would you like to be treated in this situation, or how would you wish one of your relatives to be treated. Occasionally, another touchstone which can be helpful is to ponder: 'would you treat this patient any differently if they were a VIP?' or perhaps a member of the Royal Family! One must aim to treat all patients with similar standards, to the highest possible level, as far as can be attainable.

Consultations must be carried out in an acceptable environment, which is stress-free, for both the doctor and the patient. Interruptions must be minimised and the room must be comfortable and allow the doctor and the patient to have eye contact at the same level.

I believe that it is good practice to welcome in each patient personally by shaking his or her hand. This is not only a common courtesy; I believe touching adds to the relationship between a doctor and his or her patient. We have many social taboos about touching, but in stressful circumstances, it is interesting to see that touching is widely practised. At times of great emotion, even men are known to touch each other, after going on a football or rugby field or at games of baseball or American football!

Touching acknowledges the common humanity of doctor and patient.

Occasionally, the patient wishes to bring a friend or a patient advocate. I know that many doctors become disconcerted with this but, on the whole, I have found that these people are usually highly motivated, through friendship or whatever, and both interpret and interpolate information and assist the patient in asking questions.

BREAKING BAD NEWS

Buckman[3] describes a six-step protocol about breaking bad news.

Getting the environment right corresponds to his step 1 of getting started. This means getting the physical context right and who should be there.

His step 2 is finding out how much the patient knows. It can be useful to ask the patient or his wife to state where they think things are at. This breaks the ice with social conversation and it can be a useful way of ascertaining the depth of information which the patient has. Occasionally, patients will surprise you by indicating that they are perfectly well aware of the diagnosis, having either worked it out themselves or being told by a general practitioner or an informed relative. By sensitively exploring the state of the patient's knowledge, his or her emotions can usually be discerned by their reaction: nervousness, occasionally aggression or very occasionally minimisation.

A doctor must realise that every patient has a coping strategy for bad news. This may involve guilt transference, e.g. 'Why did my doctor not send me for tests earlier?', or 'Although I am sitting here pretending to listen, I am mentally shutting out everything that you are saying' or 'I just want to get out of here as soon as possible and will do anything to cut short this interview'.

Buckman talks of his step 3 as 'finding out how much the patient wants to know'. By careful and sensitive handling, it is usually possible to talk a patient through his diagnosis, its implications and what the future holds. Information can be given a very slight spin, while maintaining honesty. It takes little imagination to pick the better way of imparting news of a positive bone scan in prostate cancer: e.g.

1. 'You are riddled with cancer Mr Jones' – obviously wrong or
2. 'I am afraid that the cancer has spread to the bone'.

Buckman's step 4 is sharing information.

Step 5 is identifying and acknowledging the patient's reaction.

Step 6 is planning and follow through.

Summary of Buckman's six steps[3]

1. Get the environment right.
2. How much does the patient know?
3. How much does the patient want to know?
4. Sharing information.
5. Identify and acknowledge the patient's reaction?
6. Planning and follow through.

The interchange of information

With the information and technology of today, patients frequently present now with sheaves of information which have been gleaned from the Internet. Some doctors find this threatening, but we must analyse why this is. Sometimes it is because we are not so up to date as we ought to be and the solution to that is obvious.

I find that, assuming one has time to deal with this situation and dialogue, this is actually useful. If you do not have enough time to deal with the patient at this particular time, I think it makes sense to reschedule an appointment when you will be able to do justice to his concerns. It would be appropriate to ask a patient to summarise his concerns. It is also helpful to look at the information which the patient has and make sure that this is useful and accurate. Unfortunately, the Internet is not peer-reviewed, and so the information which the patient has may not be considered within the mainstream of professional opinion.

Dealing with uncertainty

As modern health professionals, we must also be able to say on occasions that we do not know. If we knew everything, then clearly we would be in the wrong job. There are many things, in all forms of urological cancer, which are unknown. One way of approaching this is to say that there is uncertainty and that, in this particular circumstance, you cannot advise the patient in the way that you would normally wish to do. Patients will frequently say: 'What would you do doctor?' If you have a clear picture of what you would do (honestly) in their circumstances, then it is easy to impart this. If you do not honestly know, then it is important to say so. An approach that I find helpful is to say that there is no prior correct answer to their problems, e.g. in early prostate cancer but, between you, you can work through the information and arrive at the decision which is best for the patient.

At the end of the consultation, it is useful to summarise the decisions. In the UK the summary usually takes the form of a letter to the general practitioner (GP).

If there is confusion, an offer should be made to write down the information for the patient. A copy of the letter to the GP might in some circumstances be helpful, although a separate letter might be better.

In some practices, the interview is tape-recorded and a tape can be given to the patient. If it is clear that the patient is struggling with the information, it is worth suggesting that he go and speak it over with another person in his family or his family physician and suggesting that he might wish to discuss matters again if there is a lack of clarity. It is often possible to give patients information when they leave the clinic that they are able to read at leisure.

There are a number of telephone helplines which are available for various cancers, and there are often local area support facilities for cancer patients. It should be stressed that these are there to help the patient and that there is no compulsion to use them. Many patients find them very helpful and, equally, there are some patients who do not wish to discuss their disease (as part of their coping strategy), but the door should be left open should they change their mind.

Team work

Cancer care is now very complex and, increasingly, there is an emphasis on working within teams. This means that different members of the team may be able to give a different type of information to the patient and allows for a second opinion at an early stage, without either party feeling threatened.

Isolation

For many people, the diagnosis of cancer can isolate them either from their family or from friends, or indeed from the whole world. It is important to remember that your contract is with your patient primarily and it is their welfare that is important. As the patient's doctor you have a secondary duty to their family, friends, etc., but it is to the patient that your duty is paramount. Normally, I find it better to have all conversations directly with the patient and, if you wish to speak to relatives, that you do it in the patient's presence. This way, the patient does not feel excluded from information. It is wise to avoid conspiracy with relatives to deny information to the patient no matter how bad the news. It is up to the patient to control the flow of information. They have in all probability formed an opinion, and it may be a worse picture than that which is in reality the case. Facing death is a bleak experience and the patient has a right to face it with the support of his physician, and with the support of his family. Denial by the patient is quite a different matter.

FACING DEATH

Do not go gentle into that good night,
Old age should burn and rave at close of day;
Rage, rage against the dying of the light.
Dylan Thomas

Death is so often sanitised that, for many, it represents an ultimate betrayal by doctors ('they said it would be all right, 2 years ago'), religion and even by the patient of him or herself. Relatives may deny the impending death, or fail to come to terms with the patient's demise, as Dylan Thomas, who was wrestling with his father's impending death and reacting with anger. It is important to discuss the event in a tactful but informative way. Reassurance can be made that the mode of death should be as painless as possible. One phrase that I find helpful is to say to the patient: 'remember, we are on your side.'

Patients may often wish to see distant relatives or tidy up their affairs, and it is also wise to make the point that this can be the situation for anyone in case they face sudden death. It is better to err on the side of safety. A distant relative may be able to make a second trip, but if death is quicker than expected, no such meeting is possible.

The hospital chaplaincy can be of great assistance. Your own religious beliefs must be sublimated unless asked for directly by the patient. It is not necessary to hide genuine religious conviction, as long as it is not forced on the patient, and you may be rewarded with genuine interest. An honest answer to a direct question is the only possible one. It can be very helpful to involve the interdenominational chaplain at the patient's request.

Prognosis

Patients often ask for a prognosis. It is an answer best avoided. I know of one surgeon who confidently diagnosed a gastric cancer and gave a very short prognosis. The patient had great delight in reporting to the surgeon's clinic for the next 20 years! Unfortunately, this is seldom the case nowadays, but it is a wise doctor who avoids being too specific. An estimate in terms of 'months' or 'a matter of months' is usually sufficient.

Place of death

Patients still find hospitals and doctors threatening. Many or most patients wish to die at home. The family may not wish this usually, because of their fear of the process and a genuine feeling of inadequacy in providing nursing care. Life has become sanitised and modern families are not exposed to death, and often birth also. Facilities should be made available to allow the patient to die at home with dignity, if that is their wish. The support of the family practitioner/GP is invaluable in this.

The next of kin

It must be remembered that the relatives need support after bereavement and this is usually in the realm of the family practitioner and paramedical support services. When dealing with the bereaved, it is helpful to recognise the stages of grief that the bereaved may suffer:

Stages of grief

- Shock and disbelief – e.g. numbness
- Expressions of grief – e.g. guilt, anger and aggression
- Depression and apathy – e.g. loss of identity, lack of self-confidence
- Recovery.

PATIENT INFORMATION

Information booklets by Cancerbacup

Cancerbacup
3 Bath Place
Rivington Street
London
EC2 3JR
0800-181199 (Freeline)
www.cancerbacup.org.uk

- Coping at home
- Coping with hair loss
- Facing the challenge of advanced cancer
- Feeling better
- Controlling pain and other symptoms of cancer
- Understanding chemotherapy
- Understanding cancer of the bladder
- Understanding cancer of the kidney
- Understanding cancer of the prostate
- Understanding clinical trials
- Understanding radiotherapy
- Understanding testicular cancer

The Cancer Guide
Macmillan Cancer Relief
PO Box 7
London
W5 2GQ

Bereavement
Help the Aged
St James Walk
Clerkenwell Green
London
EC1R 0BE

Useful web sites

American Cancer Society:
http://www.cancer.org
American Urological Association:
www.auanet.org
Cancerbacup:
http://www.cancerbacup.org.uk
Cancer Research Campaign
http://wwwcrc.org.uk

National Cancer Institute, USA:
http://www.nci.nih.gov
SEER Cancer Statistics:
http://www.seer.ims.nci.nih.gov

Guide to Internet resources for cancer:
www.ncl.ac.uk/child-health/guides/clinks1.html

REFERENCES

1. Baden M. In: Artist's death: a last statement in a thesis on 'self-determination', Johnston L (ed.). New York Times, 17 June 1979, pp 1, 10
2. Szasz T. The second sin. London: Anchor Press, 1973
3. Buckman R. How to break bad news. London: Pan Books, 1992

FURTHER READING

Ader R, Cohen N, Felten D. Psychoneuro-immunology: interactions between the nervous system and the immune system. Lancet 1995; 345:99–103

Fallowfield L. Getting sad and bad news. Lancet 1993; 341:476–478

Faulkner A. When the news is bad. Cheltenham: Stanley Thornes, 1998

Penson RT, Slevin L. Communication with the cancer patient. In: Treatment of cancer, 3rd edn, Price P, Sikora K (eds). London: Chapman and Hall Medical, 1995

Phillips RH. Coping with prostate cancer. New York: Avery Publishing Group, 1994

Silverman J, Kurtz S, Draper D. Skills for communicating with patients. Oxford: Oxford University Press, 1998

Tate P. The doctor's communication handbook, 2nd edn. Oxford: Radcliffe Medical Press, 1997

13

Clinical trials and research

I have no data yet. It is a capital mistake to theorise before one has data. Insensibly one begins to twist facts to suit theories, instead of theories to suit facts.

Arthur Conan Doyle[1]

The statistical correlation does not ipso facto signify that either one is the cause or effect of the other.

John Punnett Peters[2]

GENERAL COMMENTARY

Research

For many clinicians, research is merely a hurdle to be cleared in the pursuit of a goal in a clinical career. It is almost self-evident that clinical trials are an important aspect of a clinician's work. During the preparatory phase, and indeed later, the subject of basic research comes up. Some young clinicians get excellent guidance as to what to pursue. The following Ten Commandments is a useful matrix which I use and re-read every so often to help refocus.

Ten Commandments for picking a research project[3]
1. Anticipate the results before doing the first study
2. Pick an area on the basis of the interest of the outcome
3. Look for an under-occupied niche that has potential
4. Go to talks and read papers outside your area of interest
5. Build on a theme
6. Find a balance between low-risk and high-risk projects, but always include a high-risk, high-interest project in your portfolio
7. Be prepared to pursue a project to any depth necessary
8. Differentiate yourself from your mentor
9. Do not assume that outstanding, or even good, clinical research is easier than outstanding basic research
10. Focus, focus and focus.

The main considerations of a project are:
'So what?' and
'Who cares?'

Clinical trials

At first sight, it is difficult to understand the need for a clinical trial.

Most clinicians are familiar with the discovery of penicillin: a new wonder drug had been isolated and synthesised. When it was given to patients *in extremis*, they survived when previously they would have died. It must have been extraordinarily exciting to be given such a marvellous drug, where previously there had been little which produced any effect.

Using this analogy, sceptics decide that clinical trials are unnecessary. Speaking as a surgeon, I know that many of us are responsible for small studies, and we claim to show benefit where it may not be generally applicable.

The reason that we must do clinical trials is

that, in almost every case, we are not lucky enough to be given an entirely new drug with the increased activity of penicillin. We are looking for differences or improvements in treatment between 10% and 20%, which are worth having, particularly if you are in the 10–20% of patients who benefit.

Cancer care is extraordinarily complex and each tumour may have an increasingly random behaviour pattern; it is pitting its activities against a unique genetic organism, i.e. you and me.

This concept has led to the science of pharmacogenomics. Genetic information is used to narrow down treatments to patients who are more or less likely to benefit from a particular treatment.

As a surgeon, if I am honest, I know that I tend to select the patients who I know will do well: this is part of the art of medicine, but it immediately introduces a selection bias into our treatments.

If we are able to remove lymph nodes from some of our patients, we are able to stage them – usually and unfortunately upstaging them – whereas our radiotherapy colleagues do not normally have the benefit of this super selection; thus, we immediately bias our results in the area of surgery.

To rule out this selection bias, it is necessary to randomise patients between two different treatments. It is important that this randomisation is kept as much at arms length from the individual clinicians, and agreed criteria are usually drawn up for entry into a trial.

We know that enthusiastic doctors get better results than pessimistic doctors (the patient who has had side effects from previous treatments is more likely to have trouble with a new drug and this is a patient bias). We also know that placebos can be remarkably effective treatments!

Various attempts were made to control trials to minimise these rogue results, by using a control group, random allocation of treatments or, where possible, 'blinding' of the investigators and patients.

It is important to check that the trial objectives are appropriate. For cancer patients, end points usually involve death, but occasionally surrogate end points can be used.

One final good reason for putting patients into trials is that we know that patients in trials have better results, regardless of treatment.[4]

EVIDENCE-BASED MEDICINE

In the last two decades there has been an explosion in the amount of scientific information published. We are all aware that some papers that are published are of much less weight than others.[5] It has finally been recognised that systematic reviews are required to integrate valid information and provide a basis for rational decision making. The use of explicit systematic methods in reviews limits bias and reduces random errors in an attempt to provide more reliable research from which to draw conclusions and make decisions.[6]

Meta-analysis

Meta-analysis is the use of statistical methods to summarise results of independent studies.[7]

It began to be recognised that many health care review articles were of poor scientific quality.[8,9]

The Cochrane Collaboration[10] was set up to provide reviews of health care and to disseminate these reviews. The Cochrane Collaboration set up Cochrane Methods Working Groups and Collaborative Review Groups, with the task of systematically reviewing the effects of health care within particular areas of interest. The Cochrane Centres provide training for reviewers.

The Cochrane Collaboration focuses on systematic reviews of randomised controlled trials (RCTs), since they feel that these are more likely to provide more reliable information than other studies. They have a highly stylised approach to the review of information, and systematic reviews are prepared using the following seven steps:

1. formulating the problem
2. locating and selecting studies

3. critical appraisal of studies
4. collecting data
5. analysing and presenting results
6. interpreting results
7. improving and updating reviews.

The search strategy for information is outlined with objectives, results, discussion and finally conclusions, as far as implications for practice. Where implications for research are concerned, all conflicts of interests have to be stated by the reviewers. Co-publication in peer review medical journals is acceptable but must be stated.

Methods of randomisation

Generation of random sequence:

1. computer
2. random number table
3. toss of a coin – cumbersome and non-verifiable
4. deck of cards – cumbersome and non-verifiable
5. alternation
6. other.

Zelen[11] suggested a different method of randomisation. Participants are not asked for consent to randomisation but are asked for consent to treatment. They may be told that they have already been randomised and that a particular treatment has been suggested and are they in agreement with this treatment, after the randomisation. This approach, although practical, has not met with much support from ethicists.

Concealment of allocation from doctor entering patient[12]

1. Centralised randomisation by telephone
2. Randomisation scheme controlled by pharmacy
3. Numbered or coded identical containers administered sequentially
4. On-site computer system which can only be accessed after entering the characteristics of an enrolled participant

5. Sequentially numbered, sealed, opaque envelopes
6. Sealed envelopes but not sequentially numbered or opaque
7. Alternation
8. Date of birth
9. Day of week (this method can be nonrandomised in certain circumstances. The check must be made to ensure that this is genuinely random).
10. A list of random numbers read by someone not entering patients into the trial (closed list)
11. List of random numbers read by someone entering patient into the trial (open list)
12. Other method.

Life tables

Early attempts at description of survival involved the reporting of 'average survival'.[13]

To estimate survival, one of the first methods used was to quote mean survival. These results depend upon the length of follow-up, unless all subjects have died. Occasionally, a 5-year survival time has been computed, since it is believed that in many cancers the rate of recurrence after 5 years would be very low. This is of course not very meaningful in, for example, renal cancer. In cancers at an early stage, where survival can be long, it can take too long to compute the mean survival.

Construction of life tables
Life tables involve using the data from all subjects in a study.

Median survival
This is defined as the length of follow-up when exactly 50% of the sample have died. This can be meaningful where there is a constant death rate, but can be quite misleading if the death rate is not evenly distributed throughout the years.

Survival analyses
Where adjacent curves do not overlap and there is 95% confidence that the roles do not overlap,

there is a less than 5%, i.e. $p < 0.05$, that the result has occurred by chance.

EVALUATION OF TREATMENT EFFICACY

Four standard definitions of response in solid tumours are used:
- *complete remission (CR)*: the disappearance of all tumours for a period of at least 4 weeks
- *partial remission (PR)*: tumour shrinkage to more than 50% of initial size for a period of at least 4 weeks
- *no change (NC)* or stable disease (SD)
- *progressive disease (PD)*: an increase in tumour size during treatment.

Occasionally, changes in lymph node size may be seen which are less than 50% and so these standard definitions can be modified.

Occasionally, response is measured in terms of a biochemical indicator, such as prostate-specific antigen (PSA), rather than lymph node size. When trials are reported, it is important to check which system the authors have used and whether they have used it consistently throughout their paper and also to assess whether the system they have used is appropriate, reasonable and comparable to the systems used in other treatments.

STATISTICAL ANALYSIS

Definition of odds

This is the ratio of probabilities of two mutually exclusive conditions: e.g. the probability of having a disease, divided by the probability of not having the disease.[14]

Odds ratio

The ratio of two odds. This is the odds of disease in an exposed individual and the unexposed individual. This is often used as an estimate of the relative risk in a case controlled study.[14]

Standard deviation

The standard deviation is the square root of the variance. The variance itself is the sum of squares of all individual differences of observations from the mean, divided by the number of observations. The variance and the standard deviation are the most important measures of dispersion of a series of figures in a range of observations.

The mean is the sum of all observations, divided by the number of observations. Occasionally, with large variations in numbers, the geometric mean is used (this is the antilog of the mean of the log minus the transformed data).

Statistical tests

There are numerous tests for examining differences between different statistical groups and Table 13.1 summarises some of the different tests.

A test is chosen for comparing averages of two or more samples of scores from experiments with one treatment factor.

The statistical analysis of trials is really beyond the scope of this chapter. Survival tables are usually produced by the method described by Kaplan & Meier.[16] These are essentially actuarial survival tables that are used by actuaries to plot survival in order to calculate life insurance. Survival curves are plotted, usually comparing two different treatment regimes, and a test of statistical significance is used. Maentel & Hanszel[17] described one of the first methods, and then Peto et al[18] produced the log rank test that employs a nonparametric chi-square statistic to assess the probabilities of a real statistical difference existing, i.e. one not having occurred by chance.

The p value, which is derived, quantifies the chance that a difference exists and what the chances are that any difference is real or has happened by the play of chance. The total number of deaths at each event time and their proportions in each treatment group can be calculated as the observed (O) and the expected (E). The t-statistic is the sum of:

$$(O - E)^2/E \qquad \text{for each group}$$

If the null hypothesis is true, i.e. that no

Table 13.1 Experimental design of different tests (from Kinnear & Gray[15])		
Type of data	Between subjects (independent samples)	Within subjects (related samples)
	2 samples	2 samples
Interval	Independent samples t-test	Paired samples t-test
Ordinal	Wilcoxon–Mann–Whitney test	Wilcoxon signed ranks test
		Sign test
Nominal	Chi-square	McNemar
	3 or more samples	3 or more samples
Interval	One-way ANOVA	Repeated measures ANOVA
Ordinal	Kruskal–Wallis k-sample	Friedman
Nominal	Chi-square	Cochran's Q (dichotomous nominal data only)

difference exists, then t is distributed in a similar fashion to the chi-square statistic. If two groups are compared, there is only one degree of freedom; if more than two, then the number of degrees of freedom is the number of groups minus one.

Intention to treat

Occasionally, there can be differences between 'on treatment analysis' – confined to patients who continue on randomised treatment – and an 'intention to treat analysis', which examines the outcome as if the patients had received their original randomised treatment. This latter analysis is usually given more respect, since randomised treatment may be stopped or changed for safety reasons. Intention to treat is generally interpreted as including all patients, regardless of whether they actually satisfied the entry criteria, the treatment actually received and subsequent withdrawal or deviation from the protocol. Clinical effectiveness may be overestimated if an intention to treat analysis is not done. The approach maintains treatment groups that are similar, apart from random variation. In addition, intention to treat analysis allows for noncompliance and protocol deviations by clinicians.

Key points

Key points of intention to treat are taken from Hollis & Campbell:[19]

- Intention to treat gives a pragmatic estimate of the benefit of a change in treatment policy rather than of the potential benefit in patients who receive treatment exactly as planned
- Full application of intention to treat is possible only when complete outcome data are available for all randomised subjects
- About half of all published reports of randomised controlled trials stated that intention to treat was used, but handling of deviations from randomised allocation varied widely
- Many trials had some missing data on the primary outcome variable, and methods used to deal with this were generally inadequate, potentially leading to bias
- Intention to treat analyses are often inadequately described and inadequately applied

Types of statistical error

It is a sad and published fact that statistics can be used inappropriately. There are two types of error commonly found.

Type I

A type I error is where a difference is reported but it is not a real difference: it has arisen by chance alone and is not due to treatment.

Type II

A type II error is a common problem where studies do not have enough patients enrolled to demonstrate a real difference. Thus, the study does not possess enough power to detect a real difference: i.e. one that is clinically significant. Tests are available to check for power, and good studies report it in trial design.

It is now accepted practice for 95% confidence intervals to be calculated. There is a danger of performing subgroup analysis to show differences which may not be clinically important. Where small groups are compared, the differences may occur by chance and they must be taken within the context of the entire trial.

Power

Power is the confidence with which the investigator can claim that a specified treatment benefit has not been overlooked.[20] A percentage of 80% is a realistic target.

Some examples of errors in analysis[21,22]

Definite errors
- Unpaired method for paired data
- Using a *t*-test for comparing survival times (some of which are censored)
- Use of correlation to relate change to initial value
- Comparison of *p* values
- Failure to take account of ordering of several groups
- Wrong units of analysis.

Matters of judgement
- Whether to suggest that the author adjust the analysis for potential confounding variables
- Is the rationale for categorisation of continuous variables clear?

- Are categories collapsed without adequate justification?

Poor reporting
- Failure to specify all methods used
- Wrong names for statistical methods: such as variance analysis, multivariate analysis (for multiple regression)
- Misuse of technical terms, such as quartile
- Citing nonexistent methods such as 'arc sinus transformation' and 'impaired *t*-test' (seen in published papers)
- Referring to unusual/obscure methods without explanation or reference.

Some examples of errors in design[21,22]

Definite errors
- Failure to use proper randomisation, particularly proper allocation concealment, in a controlled trial
- Use of an inappropriate control group
- Use of a crossover design for a study of a condition that can be cured, such as infertility
- Failure to anticipate regression to the mean.

Matters of judgement
- Is the sample size large enough?
- Is the response rate adequate?

Poor reporting
- Study aims not stated
- Justification of sample size not given
- In a controlled trial, method of randomisation not stated.

Some examples of errors in interpretation[21,22]

Definite errors
- Failure to consider confidence interval when interpreting nonsignificant (NS) difference, especially in a small study
- Drawing conclusions about causation from an observed association
- Interpreting a poor study as if it were a

good study (e.g. a small study as a large study, a nonrandomised study as a randomised study).

Matters of judgement
- Would results be better in a table or figure?
- Have the authors taken adequate account of possible sources of bias?
- How should multiplicity be handled (e.g. multiple time points or multiple groups)?
- Is there over-reliance on p values?

Poor reporting
- Discussion of analyses not included in the paper
- Drawing conclusions not supported by the study data.

Some examples of errors in presentation[21,22]

Definite errors
- Giving standard error instead of standard deviation to describe data
- Pie charts to show the distribution of continuous variables
- Results given only as p values
- Confidence intervals given for each group, rather than for the contrast
- Use of scale changes or breaks in histograms
- Failure to show all points in scatter diagrams.

Matters of judgement
- Would the data be better in a table or a figure?
- Should we expect authors to have considered (and commented on) goodness of fit?

Poor reporting
- Numerical results given to too many or, occasionally, to too few decimal places
- r or chi-square values to too many decimal places
- 'p = NS', 'p = 0.0000', etc.
- Reference to 'nonparametric data'
- Tables that do not add up, or which do not agree with each other.

Table 13.2 lists items that should be included in reports of randomised trials.

Publication bias

Editors and reviewers tend to prefer studies which show a positive result. It is much more difficult to get a negative study published.[24] To some extent, this can be addressed by structured literature reviews which compare the results of negative studies that may be more likely to have been published in more obscure and less well-read journals. Most clinicians know the reviewers that they respect and will follow their judgement. A checklist is shown in Box 13.1.

Heading	Subheading	Descriptor
Table 13.2	**Items that should be included in reports of randomised trials (reproduced from Begg et al[23])**	
Title		Identify the study as a randomised trial
Abstract		Use a structured format
Introduction		State prospectively defined hypothesis, clinical objectives and planned subgroup or cohort analyses
Methods	Protocol	Describe: • planned study population, together with inclusion or exclusion criteria • planned interventions and their timing • primary and secondary outcome measure(s) and the minimum important difference(s), and indicate how the target sample size was projected • rationale and methods for statistical analyses, detailing main comparative analyses and whether they were completed on an intention to treat basis • prospectively defined stopping rules (if warranted)
	Assignment	Describe: • unit of randomisation (e.g. individual, cluster, geographic) • method used to generate the allocation schedule • method of allocation concealment and timing of assignment • method to separate the generator from the executor of assignment
	Masking (blinding)	Describe: • mechanism (e.g. capsules, tablets) • similarity of treatment characteristics (e.g. appearance, taste) • allocation schedule control (location of code during trial and when broken) • evidence for successful blinding among participants, person doing intervention, outcome assessors and data analysts
Results	Participant flow and follow-up	Provide a trial profile, summarising participant flow, numbers and timing, of randomisation assignment, interventions and measurements for each randomised group
	Analysis	• State estimated effect of intervention on primary and secondary outcomes, measures, including a point estimate and measure of precision (confidence interval) • State results in absolute numbers when feasible (e.g., 10/20, not 50%) • Present summary data and appropriate descriptive and interferential statistics in sufficient detail to permit alternative analyses and replication • Describe prognostic variables by treatment group and any attempt to adjust for them • Describe protocol deviations from the study as planned; together with the reasons
Discussion		• State specific interpretation of study findings, including sources of bias and imprecision (internal validity) and discussion of external validity, including appropriate quantitative measures when possible • State general interpretation of the data in light of the totality of the available evidence

DRUG DEVELOPMENT

Each pharmaceutical company tests thousands of compounds every year in an attempt to find one which has therapeutic promise. The process may involve screening of synthetic chemicals and natural products from plants, microbes and yeasts. Occasionally, drugs, which were destined for one use, are found to be far better for others, e.g. sildenafil (Viagra).

Once a drug has been identified, it goes through extensive animal pharmacology studies, to identify a likely human dosage. Pharmacokinetic data such as absorption distribution, metabolism and excretion will be ascertained in animals. The toxicology of the drug is also obtained in animals.

After an extensive period of evaluation, drugs are then entered into clinical development. This occurs in five phases.[25,26]

Phase 1
Clinical pharmacology in normal volunteers. This is done to establish tolerated doses and generate pharmacokinetic and safety data in humans. Cytotoxic drugs are not subjected to phase 1 testing, however, for obvious reasons.

Phase 2
Patients are treated to investigate the kinetics of the drug, to provide some evidence of efficacy and also to allow dose ranging.

Phase 3
Once efficacy has been established, formal therapeutic trials and evidence of safety can be obtained. At this stage, preclinical pharmaceutical and clinical data will be submitted for a license to sell the drug.

Phase 4
Post-marketing surveillance, which is necessary to establish long-term safety.

Phase 5
Comparison of the drug with other similar compounds, and also exploration of new indications for the drug.

In the United States, the Food and Drug Administration (FDA) introduced drug regulatory laws in 1937. Europe introduced them in 1961, after the thalidomide tragedy.

In the UK, a Clinical Trials Certificate (CTC) or a Clinical Trials Exemption Certificate (CTX) is needed.

It is only after all data have been formally reviewed that a product license is granted.

A degree of harmonisation have been produced that allows data from Europe and the United States to be interchangeable. This has been due to the introduction of standard good laboratory practices (GLP) and good clinical practices (GCP) by the European Agencies and the US FDA.

REFERENCES

1. Doyle AC. A scandal in Bohemia. Republished in: Sherlock Holmes, The complete short stories. London: Chancellor Press, 1987
2. Peters JP. Some remarks on renal disease. Yale J Biol Med 1953; 26:179–190
3. Ronald C, Kahn MD. Picking a research problem. N Engl J Med 1994; 21:1530–1533
4. Stiller CA. Centralized therapy, entry to trials and survival. Br J Cancer 1994; 70:352–362
5. Oxman AD, Guyatt GH. The science of reviewing research. Ann NY Acad Sci 1993; 703:125–133
6. Mulrow CD. Rationale for systematic reviews. Br Med J 1994; 309(6954):597–599
7. Antman EM, Lau J, Kupelnick B, Mosteller F, Chalmers TC. A comparison of results of meta-analyses of randomized control trials and recommendations of clinical experts. Treatments of myocardial infarction. JAMA 1992; 268(2): 240–248
8. Kleijnen J, Gotzsche PC, Kunz RA, et al. Chalmers I, Maynard A, editors. Non-random reflections on health care research: on the 25th anniversary of Archie Cochrane's effectiveness and efficiency. London: BMJ Publishers, So what's so special about randomization?
9. Moher D, Jadad AR, Nichol G, Penman M, Tugwell T, Walsh S. Assessing the quality of randomized controlled trials: an annotated bibliography of scales and checklists. Controlled Clin Trials 1995; 16(1):62–73
10. Chalmers I. The Cochrane Collaboration: preparing, maintaining and disseminating systematic reviews of the effects of health care. Ann NY Acad Sci 1993; 703:156–165
11. Zelen M. A new design for randomized clinical trials. N Engl J Med 1979; 300:1242–1245
12. Mathews DE, Farewell V. Using and understanding medical statistics. New York: Karger, 1985
13. Philips RKS. Life tables in principles of surgical research. In: Principles of surgical research, Massie ART, Taylor KM, Calman JS (eds). London: Wright, 1989
14. Petrie A, Sabin C. Medical statistics at a glance. Oxford: Blackwells Science, 2000
15. Kinnear PR, Gray CD. SPSS for Windows made simple, 2nd edn, Choosing a statistical test. Psychology Press, East Sussex, 1997; 5:110
16. Kaplan EL, Meier P. Nonparametric estimation from incomplete observations. J R Statist Soc A 1958; 53:457–481
17. Maentel N, Hanszel W. Statistical aspects of the analysis of data from retrospective studies of disease. J Natl Cancer Inst 1959; 22:719–748
18. Peto R, Pike MC, Armitage P, et al. Design and analysis of randomized clinical trials requiring prolonged observation of each patient. II. Analysis and examples. Br J Cancer 1977; 35:1–39
19. Hollis S, Campbell F. What is meant by intention to treat analysis? Survey of published randomised controlled trials. Br Med J 1999; 319: 670–674
20. Gore SM, Altman DG. Statistics in practice. London: BMJ Books, 1982
21. Altman DG. Statistical reviewing for medical journals. Stat Med 1998; 17:2662–2676
22. Godlee F, Jefferson T. Peer review in health statistics. London: BMJ Books, 1999
23. Begg C, Cho M, Eastwood S, et al. Improving the quality of reporting of randomized controlled trials: the CONSORT statement. JAMA 1966; 276:637–639
24. Berlin JA, Begg CB, Louis TA. An assessment of publication bias using sample of published clinical trials. J Am Stat Assoc 1989; 84:381–392
25. Oxman AD. Checklists for review articles. Br Med J 1994; 309(6955):648–651
26. Harry J, McInnes G, Waller P, Ramsay L, Yeo W. Symposium. Prescribers J 1991; 31(6):219–257

FURTHER READING

General statistics

Armitage P. Statistical methods in medical research. Oxford: Blackwell, 1971

Chatellier G, Zapletal E, Lemaitre D, Menard J, Degoulet P. The number needed to treat: a clinically useful nomogram in its proper context. Br Med J 1996; 312:426–429

Eddy DM. Anatomy of a decision. JAMA 1990; 263(3):441–443

Hill AB. Principles of medical statistics, 9th edn. London: Lancet, 1971:312–320

Light RJ, Smith PV. Accumulating evidence: procedures for resolving contradictions among different research studies. Harv Educ Rev 1971; 41: 429–471

Mulrow CD. The medical review article: state of the science. Ann Intern Med 1987; 106(3):485–488

Oxman AD, Guyatt GH. Guidelines for reading literature reviews. Can Med Assoc J 1988; 138(8):697–703

General

Begg CB, Berlin JA. Publication bias and dissemination of clinical research. J Natl Cancer Inst 1989; 81(2):107–115

Feinstein AR, Horwitz RI. Double standards, scientific methods, and epidemiological research. N Engl J Med 1982; 307(26):1611–1617

Fleiss JL. Statistical methods for rates and proportions, 2nd edn. New York: John Wiley and Sons, 1981

Lancet. Making clinical trialists register. Lancet 1991; 338:244–245

Levine M, Walter S, Lee H, Haines T, Holbrook A, Moyer V. User's guides to the medical literature, IV. How to use an article about harm. Evidence-Based Medicine Working Group. JAMA 1994; 271(20):1615–1619

Oxman AD, Cook DJ, Guyatt GH. Users' guides to the medical literature, VI. How to use an overview. Evidence-Based Medicine Working Group. JAMA 1994; 272(17):1367–1371

Trials

Chalmers TC, Celano P, Sacks HS, Smith H Jr. Bias in treatment assignment in controlled clinical trials.

N Engl J Med 1983; 309(22):1358–1361

Jadad AR, Moore RA, Carroll D, et al. Assessing the quality of reports of randomized clinical trials: Is blinding necessary? Controlled Clin Trials 1996; 17:1–12

Oxman AD, Guyatt GH. A consumer's guide to subgroup analyses. Ann Intern Med 1992; 116(1):78–84

Peto R, Pike MC, Armitage P, et al. Design and analysis of randomized clinical trials requiring prolonged observation of each patient. I. Introduction and design. Br J Cancer 1976; 34: 585–612

Sacks HS, Chalmers TC, Smith H. Randomized versus historical controls for clinical trials. Am J Med 1982; 72:233–240

Silverman WA, Altman DG. Patients' preferences and randomised trials. Lancet 1996; 347:171–174

Wilt TJ. Can randomised treatment trials in early stage prostate cancer be completed? Clin Oncol 1998; 10(3):141–143

Meta-analysis

Berlin JA, Laird NM, Sacks HS, Chalmers TC. A comparison of statistical methods for combining event rates from clinical trials. Stat Med 1989; 8(2):141–151

Eddy DM, Hasselblad V, Shachter R. An introduction to a Bayesian method for meta-analyses: the confidence profile method. Med Decis Making 1990; 10(1):15–23

Hedges LV, Olkin I. Statistical methods for meta-analysis. Orlando: Academic Press, 1985

L'Abbe KA, Detsky AS, O'Rouke K. Meta-analysis in clinical research. Ann Intern Med 1987; 107(2):224–233

Sacks HS, Berrier J, Reitman D, Ancona-Berk VA, Chalmers TC. Meta-analyses of randomised controlled trials. N Engl J Med 1987; 316(8):450–455

Thacker SB. Meta-analysis: a quantitative approach to research integration. JAMA 1988; 259(11):1685–1689

Thompson SG, Pocock SJ. Can meta-analyses be trusted? Lancet 1991; 338(8775):1127–1130

Cochrane

Cochrane Collaboration, editor. Cochrane Database of Systematic Reviews. 1996; Oxford: Update Software. Updated quarterly. Available from:

BMJ Publishing Group, London

Mulrow CD, Oxman A. How to conduct a Cochrane Systematic Review. San Antonio Cochrane Collaboration, September 1997, Version 3.02

NHS Centre for Reviews and Dissemination, ed. Database of Abstracts of Reviews of Effectiveness. 1996; Oxford: Update Software. Updated quarterly. Available from: BMJ Publishing Group, London

Oxman AD, Guyatt GH. Guidelines for reading literature reviews. Can Med Assoc J 1988; 138(8):697–703

Stewart LA, Clarke M, for the Cochrane Collaboration Working Group on meta-analyses using individual patient data. Practical methodology of meta-analyses (overviews) using updated individual patient data. Stat Med 1995; 14:2057–2079

General bibliography

Belldegrun A, Kirby R, Oliver T. New perspectives in prostate cancer. Oxford: Isis Medical Media, 1998

Bostwick D. Uropathology. The urologic clinics of North America. Philadelphia: WB Saunders, 1999

Hermanek P, Hutter RVP, Sobin LH, Wagner G, Wittekind CH. TNM atlas, 4th edn. Union International Centre Le Cancer: Springer, 1997

Parkin DM, Whelan SL, Ferlay J, Raymond L, Young J. Cancer incidence in five continents, Vol. VII. Lyon: IARC Scientific Publications, No 143, 1997

Price P, Sikora K. Treatment of cancer, 3rd edn. London: Chapman and Hall, 1995

Raghavan DK, Scher HI, Leibel SA, Lange P (eds). Principles & practice of genitourinary oncology. Philadelphia: Lippincott, 1997

Walsh PC, Retik AB, Vaughan ED, Wein AJ (eds). Campbell's urology, 7th edn. Philadelphia: WB Saunders, 1997

Appendix A

Nomogram for calculation of trial sizes

Nomogram to determine numbers need for clinical trials. Reproduced with permission from BMJ publications.

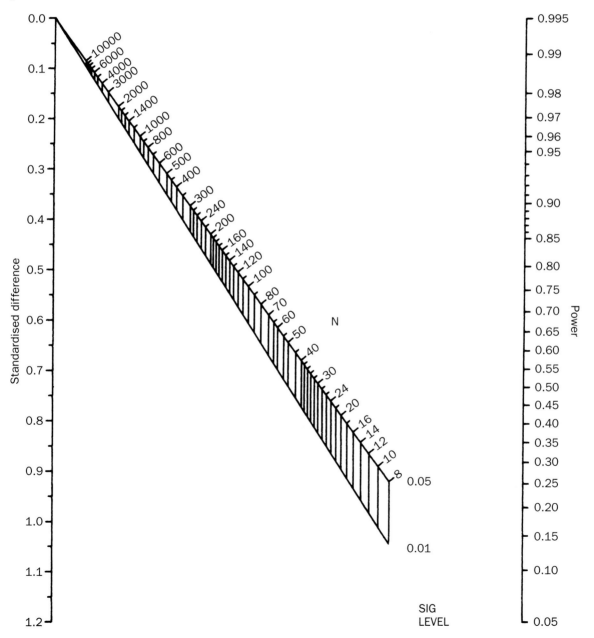

Appendix B

Performance status: WHO and ECOG

WHO PERFORMANCE STATUS: CLINICAL PERFORMANCE STATUS

0   Able to carry out all normal activity without restriction.
1   Restricted in physically strenuous activity but ambulatory and able to carry out light work.
2   Ambulatory and capable of all self-care but unable to carry out any work; up and about more than 50% of waking hours.
3   Capable only of limited self-care; confined to bed or chair more than 50% of waking hours.
4   Completely disabled; cannot carry out any self-care; totally confined to bed or chair.

ECOG PERFORMANCE STATUS

0   Fully active, able to carry on all pre-disease performance without restriction.
1   Restricted in physically strenuous activity but ambulatory and able to carry out work of a light or sedentary nature, e.g. light housework, office work.
2   Ambulatory and capable of all self-care but unable to carry out any work activities. Up and about more than 50% of waking hours.
3   Capable of only limited self-care, confined to bed or chair more than 50% of waking hours.
4   Completely disabled. Cannot carry on any self-care. Totally confined to bed or chair.
5   Dead.

Appendix C

Declaration of Helsinki (Revision 1996)

These are recommendations guiding physicians in biochemical research involving human subjects.

INTRODUCTION

It is the mission of the physician to safeguard the health of the people. His or her knowledge and conscience are dedicated to the fulfillment of this mission.

The Declaration of Geneva of the World Medical Association binds the physician with the words: 'The health of my patient will be my first consideration', and the International Code of Medical Ethics declares that 'A physician shall act only in the patient's interest when providing medical care which might have the effect of weakening the physical and mental condition of the patient'.

The purpose of biomedical research involving human subjects must be to improve diagnostic, therapeutic and prophylactic procedures and the understanding of the aetiology and pathogenesis of disease.

In current medical practice, most diagnostic, therapeutic or prophylactic procedures involve hazards. This applies especially to biomedical research. Medical progress is based on research, which ultimately must rest in part on experimentation involving human subjects.

In the field of biomedical research a fundamental distinction must be recognised between medical research – in which the aim is essentially diagnostic or therapeutic for a patient – and medical research, the essential object of which is purely scientific, without implying direct diagnostic or therapeutic value to the person subjected to the research.

Special caution must be exercised in the conduct of research which may affect the environment, and the welfare of animals used for research must be respected.

Because it is essential that the results of laboratory experiments be applied to human beings to further scientific knowledge and to help suffering humanity, the World Medical Association has prepared the following recommendations as a guide to every physician in biomedical research involving human subjects. They should be kept under review in the future. It must be stressed that the standards as drafted are only a guide to physicians all over the world. Physicians are not relieved from criminal, civil and ethical responsibilities under the laws of their own countries.

BASIC PRINCIPLES

1. Biomedical research involving human subjects must conform to generally accepted scientific principles and should be based on adequately performed laboratory and animal experimentation and on a thorough knowledge of the scientific tradition.

2. The design and performance of each experimental procedure involving human subjects should be clearly formulated in an experimental protocol which should be transmitted for consideration, comment and guidance to a specially appointed committee independent of the investigator and the sponsor provided that this independent committee is in conformity with the laws and regulations of the country in which the

research experiment is performed.

3. Biomedical research involving human subjects should be conducted only by scientifically qualified persons and under the supervision of a clinically competent medical person. The responsibility for the human subject must always rest with a medically qualified person and never rest on the subject of the research, even though the subject has given his or her consent.

4. Biomedical research involving human subjects cannot legitimately be carried out unless the importance of the objective is in proportion to the inherent risk to the subject.

5. Every biomedical research project involving human beings should be preceded by careful assessment of predictable risks in comparison with foreseeable benefits to the subject or to others. Concern for the interests of the subject must always prevail over the interests of science and society.

6. The right of the research subject to safeguard his or her integrity must always be respected. Every precaution should be taken to respect the privacy of the subject and to minimise the impact of the study on the subject's physical and mental integrity and on the personality of the subject.

7. Physicians should abstain from engaging in research projects involving human subjects unless they are satisfied that the hazards involved are believed to be predictable. Physicians should cease any investigation if the hazards are found to outweigh the potential benefits.

8. In publication of the results of his or her research, the physician is obliged to preserve the accuracy of the results. Reports of experimentation not in accordance with the principles laid down in this Declaration should not be accepted for publication.

9. In any research on human beings, each potential subject must be adequately informed of the aims, methods, anticipated benefits and potential hazards of the study and the discomfort it may entail. He or she should be informed that he or she is at liberty to abstain from participation in the study and that he or she is free to withdraw his or her consent to participation at any time. The physicians should then obtain the subject's freely-given informed consent, preferably in writing.

10. When obtaining informed consent for the research project the physician should be particularly cautious if the subject is in a dependent relationship to him or her or may consent under duress. In that case the informed consent should be obtained by a physician who is not engaged in the investigation and who is completely independent of this official relationship.

11. In case of legal incompetence, informed consent should be obtained from the legal guardian in accordance with national legislation. Where physical or mental incapacity make it impossible to obtain informed consent, or when the subject is a minor, permission from the responsible relative replaces that of the subject in accordance with national legislation. Whenever the minor child is in fact able to give a consent, the minor's consent must be obtained in addition to the consent of the minor's legal guardian.

12. The research protocol should always contain a statement of the ethical considerations involved and should indicate that the principles enunciated in the present Declaration are complied with.

MEDICAL RESEARCH COMBINED WITH PROFESSIONAL CARE (CLINICAL RESEARCH)

1. In the treatment of the sick person, the physician must be free to use a new diagnostic and therapeutic measure, if in his or her judgement it offers hope of saving life, re-establishing health or alleviating suffering.

2. The potential benefits, hazards and discomfort of a new method should be weighed against the advantages of the best current diagnostic and therapeutic methods.

3. In any medical study, every patient –

including those of a control group, if any – should be assured of the best proven diagnostic and therapeutic methods. This does not exclude the use of inert placebo in studies where no proven diagnostic or therapeutic method exists.

4. The refusal of the patient to participate in a study must never interfere with the physician–patient relationship.

5. If the physician considers it essential not to obtain informed consent, the specific reasons for this proposal should be stated in the experimental protocol for transmission to the independent committee.

6. The physician can combine medical research with professional care, the objective being the acquisition of new medical knowledge, only to the extent that medical research is justified by its potential diagnostic or therapeutic value for the patient.

NON-THERAPEUTIC BIOMEDICAL RESEARCH INVOLVING HUMAN SUBJECTS (NON-CLINICAL BIOMEDICAL RESEARCH)

1. In the purely scientific application of medical research carried out on a human being, it is the duty of the physician to remain the protector of the life and health of that person on whom biomedical research is being carried out.

2. The subjects should be volunteers – either healthy persons or patients for whom the experimental design is not related to the patient's illness.

3. The investigator or the investigating team should discontinue the research if in his/her or their judgement it may, if continued, be harmful to the individual.

4. In research on man, the interest of science and society should never take precedence over considerations related to the well-being of the subject.

Appendix D

ASA grades

ASA1 The patient has no organic, physiological, biochemical or psychiatric disturbance. The pathological process for which operation is to be performed is localised and does not entail a systemic disturbance.

ASA2 Mild to moderate systemic disturbance caused by either the condition to be treated surgically or by other pathophysiological process.

ASA3 Severe systemic disturbance of disease from whatever cause, even though it may not be possible to define the degree of disability with finality.

ASA4 Severe systemic disorders that are already life threatening, not always correctable by operation.

ASA5 The moribund patient who has little chance of survival but is submitted to operation in desperation.

Appendix E

Guidelines on disposal of cytotoxic waste

MANAGEMENT OF SPILLAGE OF A CYTOTOXIC MEDICINE

A cytotoxic spillage kit must be available in every location where cytotoxic agents are handled, including patient's homes.

Spills and breakages must be cleared up immediately. If a spillage occurs, the following procedure should be followed:

- Before dealing with a spillage, put on two pairs of gloves and an apron.
- Liquids should be absorbed with absorbent paper towels.
- Hard surfaces should then be washed thoroughly with copious amounts of cold soapy water and dried with paper towels.
- If spillage is on clothing, the items should be removed as quickly as possible and washed separately from other clothing in cold soapy water.
- If eyes are contaminated, immediate irrigation should be carried out and medical help sought.
- Any bed linen affected should be changed and washed in cold soapy water. Mattress and furnishings should be cleaned with cold soapy water.
- All clean-up materials must be placed in two waste bags and sealed by knotting each bag. The bag should be placed in the sharps bin marked 'cytotoxic waste' for disposal.
- All incidents involving spillage or direct contact with a cytotoxic medicine or any local or systemic symptoms occurring after handling such a medicine must be reported to the Nurse Manager, and Trust Risk Manager. An Incident Record Form must be completed.

- A copy of the completed incidence form should be sent to the Medicines Unit or similar.

DISPOSAL OF CYTOTOXIC WASTE

Sharps

All sharps (needles, scalpels and any similar metal parts), with their associated syringe bodies, that have been used for treatment with cytotoxic drugs, shall be placed in a 6-litre sharps bin, obtainable from your normal supplies point, or via requisition from Central Stores.

Cytotoxic drugs containers

Cytotoxic drugs containers, e.g. infusion bag with their associated lines (but with sharps detached) that have been part of cytotoxic treatment, shall be double wrapped prior to being placed in a 6- or 12-litre sharps bin, obtainable from your normal supplies point or via requisition from Central Stores. (Double wrapping is placing waste in two yellow or clear bags, each of which is sealed with a knot – to prevent spillage.)

General

All sharps bins (as detailed above) must be sealed, the bin label completed to include patient name and address, by the Community

Nurse, and marked with an indelible ink marker: 'CYTOTOXIC WASTE'.

The Community Nurse must take the sharps bins back to base and store safely, securely and separately from any other clinical waste. (Cytotoxic waste is subject to the requirements of the Special Waste Regulations: 1996 in the UK.)

- UNDER NO CIRCUMSTANCES SHOULD ANY CYTOTOXIC WASTE SHARPS BINS BE PUT INTO BAGS
- UNDER NO CIRCUMSTANCES SHALL ANY CYTOTOXIC WASTE BE PUT INTO THE NORMAL 'ORANGE' STREAM CLINICAL WASTE SYSTEM

Appendix F

Partin's tables in prostate cancer

Partin's tables in prostate cancer are given for different prostate-specific antigen (PSA) levels in Tables A1–A4.

Table A1 Clinical stage: PSA 0–4.0 ng/ml

Gleason score	T1a	T1b	T1c	T2a	T2b	T2c	T3a
Organ-confined disease							
2–4	90 (84–95)	80 (72–86)	89 (86–92)	81 (75–86)	72 (65–79)	77 (69–83)	–
5	82 (73–90)	66 (57–73)	81 (76–84)	68 (63–72)	57 (50–62)	62 (55–69)	40 (26–53)
6	78 (68–88)	61 (52–69)	78 (74–81)	64 (59–68)	52 (46–57)	57 (51–64)	35 (22–48)
7	–	43 (34–53)	63 (58–68)	47 (41–52)	34 (29–39)	38 (32–45)	19 (11–29)
8–10	–	31 (20–43)	52 (41–62)	36 (27–45)	24 (17–32)	27 (18–36)	–
Established capsular penetration							
2–4	9 (4–15)	19 (13–26)	10 (7–14)	18 (13–23)	25 (19–32)	21 (14–28)	–
5	17 (9–26)	32 (24–40)	18 (15–22)	30 (26–35)	40 (34–46)	34 (27–40)	51 (38–65)
6	19 (11–29)	35 (27–43)	21 (18–25)	34 (30–38)	43 (38–48)	37 (31–43)	53 (41–65)
7	–	44 (35–54)	31 (26–36)	45 (40–50)	51 (46–57)	45 (38–52)	52 (40–63)
8–10	–	43 (32–56)	34 (27–44)	47 (38–56)	48 (40–57)	42 (33–52)	–
Seminal vesicle involvement							
2–4	0 (0–2)	1 (0–3)	1 (0–1)	1 (0–2)	2 (1–5)	2 (1–5)	–
5	1 (0–3)	2 (0–4)	1 (1–2)	2 (1–3)	3 (2–4)	3 (2–6)	7 (3–14)
6	1 (0–3)	2 (0–4)	1 (1–2)	2 (1–3)	3 (2–4)	4 (2–5)	7 (4–13)
7	–	6 (1–13)	4 (2–7)	6 (4–9)	10 (6–14)	12 (7–17)	19 (10–31)
8–10	–	11 (2–23)	9 (5–16)	12 (7–19)	17 (11–25)	21 (12–31)	–

Numbers represent % predictive probability (95% confidence interval).
Adapted from Partin AW et al. JAMA 1997; 277:1445–1451.

Table A2 Clinical stage: PSA 4.1–10.0 ng/ml

Gleason score	T1a	T1b	T1c	T2a	T2b	T2c	T3a
Organ-confined disease							
2–4	84 (75–92)	70 (60–79)	83 (78–88)	71 (64–78)	61 (52–69)	66 (57–74)	43 (27–58)
5	72 (60–85)	53 (44–63)	71 (67–75)	55 (51–60)	43 (38–49)	49 (42–55)	27 (17–39)
6	67 (55–82)	47 (38–57)	67 (64–70)	51 (47–54)	38 (34–43)	43 (38–49)	23 (14–34)
7	49 (34–68)	29 (21–38)	49 (45–54)	33 (29–38)	22 (18–26)	25 (20–30)	11 (6–17)
8–10	35 (18–62)	18 (11–28)	37 (28–46)	23 (16–31)	14 (9–19)	15 (10–22)	6 (3–10)
Established capsular penetration							
2–4	14 (7–23)	27 (18–37)	15 (11–20)	26 (19–33)	35 (26–43)	29 (21–37)	44 (30–59)
5	25 (14–36)	42 (32–51)	27 (23–30)	41 (36–46)	50 (45–55)	43 (37–50)	57 (46–68)
6	27 (15–39)	44 (35–53)	30 (27–33)	44 (41–48)	52 (48–56)	46 (40–51)	57 (47–67)
7	36 (20–51)	48 (38–60)	40 (35–44)	52 (48–57)	54 (49–59)	48 (42–54)	48 (37–58)
8–10	34 (17–58)	42 (28–57)	40 (33–49)	49 (42–57)	46 (39–53)	40 (31–48)	34 (24–46)
Seminal vesicle involvement							
2–4	1 (0–4)	2 (0–6)	1 (0–3)	2 (1–5)	4 (1–9)	5 (1–10)	10 (3–23)
5	2 (0–5)	3 (1–7)	2 (1–3)	3 (2–5)	5 (3–8)	6 (4–10)	12 (6–20)
6	2 (0–6)	3 (1–6)	2 (2–3)	3 (2–4)	5 (4–7)	8 (4–9)	11 (6–18)
7	6 (0–19)	9 (2–18)	8 (5–11)	10 (8–13)	15 (11–19)	18 (13–24)	26 (17–36)
8–10	10 (0–34)	15 (4–29)	15 (10–22)	19 (13–26)	24 (17–31)	28 (20–37)	35 (23–48)

Numbers represent % predictive probability (95% confidence interval).
Adapted from Partin AW et al. JAMA 1997; 277:1445–1451.

Table A3   Clinical stage: PSA 10.1–20.0 ng/ml

Gleason score	T1a	T1b	T1c	T2a	T2b	T2c	T3a
Organ-confined disease							
2–4	76 (65–88)	58 (46–69)	75 (68–82)	60 (52–70)	48 (39–58)	53 (42–64)	–
5	61 (47–78)	40 (31–50)	60 (54–65)	43 (38–49)	32 (26–37)	36 (29–43)	18 (10–27)
6	–	33 (25–42)	55 (51–59)	38 (34–43)	26 (23–31)	31 (25–37)	14 (8–22)
7	33 (19–57)	17 (11–24)	35 (31–40)	22 (18–26)	13 (11–16)	15 (11–19)	6 (3–10)
8–10	–	9 (5–16)	23 (16–32)	14 (9–19)	7 (5–11)	8 (5–12)	3 (1–5)
Established capsular penetration							
2–4	20 (10–32)	36 (26–46)	22 (16–29)	35 (26–43)	43 (34–53)	37 (27–47)	–
5	33 (18–47)	50 (39–59)	35 (30–40)	50 (45–56)	57 (51–63)	51 (43–57)	59 (47–69)
6	–	49 (38–59)	38 (34–42)	52 (48–57)	57 (51–62)	50 (44–57)	54 (44–64)
7	38 (18–61)	46 (34–60)	45 (40–50)	55 (50–60)	51 (45–57)	45 (39–52)	40 (30–50)
8–10	–	33 (21–51)	40 (33–49)	46 (38–55)	38 (30–47)	33 (24–42)	26 (17–37)
Seminal vesicle involvement							
2–4	2 (0–7)	4 (1–10)	2 (1–5)	4 (1–8)	7 (2–14)	8 (2–16)	–
5	3 (0–9)	5 (1–10)	3 (2–5)	5 (3–8)	8 (5–11)	9 (6–15)	15 (8–25)
6	–	4 (1–9)	4 (3–5)	5 (3–7)	7 (5–10)	9 (6–13)	14 (8–21)
7	8 (0–28)	11 (3–22)	12 (8–16)	14 (10–19)	18 (13–24)	22 (16–29)	28 (18–39)
8–10	–	15 (4–32)	20 (13–28)	22 (15–31)	25 (18–34)	30 (21–40)	34 (21–47)

Numbers represent % predictive probability (95% confidence interval).
Adapted from Partin AW et al. JAMA 1997; 277:1445–1451.

Table A4 Clinical stage: PSA > 20.0 ng/ml

Gleason score	T1a	T1b	T1c	T2a	T2b	T2c	T3a
Organ-confined disease							
2–4	–	38 (26–52)	58 (46–68)	41 (31–52)	29 (20–40)	–	–
5	–	23 (15–32)	40 (32–49)	26 (19–33)	17 (12–22)	19 (14–26)	8 (4–14)
6	–	17 (11–25)	35 (27–42)	22 (16–27)	13 (10–17)	15 (11–20)	6 (3–10)
7	–	–	18 (13–23)	10 (7–14)	5 (4–8)	6 (4–9)	2 (1–4)
8–10	–	3 (2–7)	10 (6–16)	5 (3–9)	3 (2–4)	3 (2–5)	1 (0–2)
Established capsular penetration							
2–4	–	47 (33–61)	34 (24–44)	48 (36–58)	52 (39–65)	–	–
5	–	57 (44–68)	48 (40–56)	60 (52–68)	61 (53–69)	55 (46–64)	54 (40–67)
6	–	51 (37–64)	49 (43–56)	60 (53–66)	57 (50–64)	51 (43–59)	46 (34–58)
7	–	–	46 (39–54)	51 (44–58)	43 (35–50)	37 (29–45)	29 (19–40)
8–10	–	24 (13–42)	34 (27–45)	37 (28–48)	28 (20–37)	23 (16–31)	17 (11–26)
Seminal vesicle involvement							
2–4	–	9 (1–22)	7 (2–15)	10 (3–20)	14 (4–29)	–	–
5	–	10 (2–21)	9 (5–14)	11 (6–17)	15 (9–23)	19 (11–28)	26 (14–41)
6	–	8 (2–17)	8 (6–12)	10 (7–15)	13 (9–19)	17 (11–24)	21 (13–33)
7	–	–	22 (15–28)	24 (17–32)	27 (20–34)	32 (24–42)	36 (25–49)
8–10	–	20 (6–43)	31 (21–42)	33 (22–45)	33 (22–45)	38 (26–51)	40 (25–55)

Numbers represent % predictive probability (95% confidence interval).
Adapted from Partin AW et al. JAMA 1997; 277:1445–1451.

Appendix G

Dosage of drugs used in prostate cancer

Information on drugs used in prostate cancer is given in Table A5. Remember to consult drug literature for contraindications, side effects and dosage modification in elderly patients.

Table A5 Drugs used in prostate cancer			
Drug (generic)	**Drug (trade name)**	**Form**	**Dose**
Bicalutamide	Casodex	Tablets	150 mg once daily
Cyproterone acetate	Cyproterone acetate, Cyprostat	Tablets	100 mg three times a day
Flutamide	Flutamide, Drogenil	Tablets	250 mg three times a day
Goserelin	Zoladex	Subcutaneous injection	3.6 mg every 28 days
		Subcutaneous injection	10.8 mg every 12 weeks
Leuprorelin acetate	Prostap	Subcutaneous injection	3.75 mg every month
		Subcutaneous injection	10.8 mg every 12 weeks

Index